I0762405

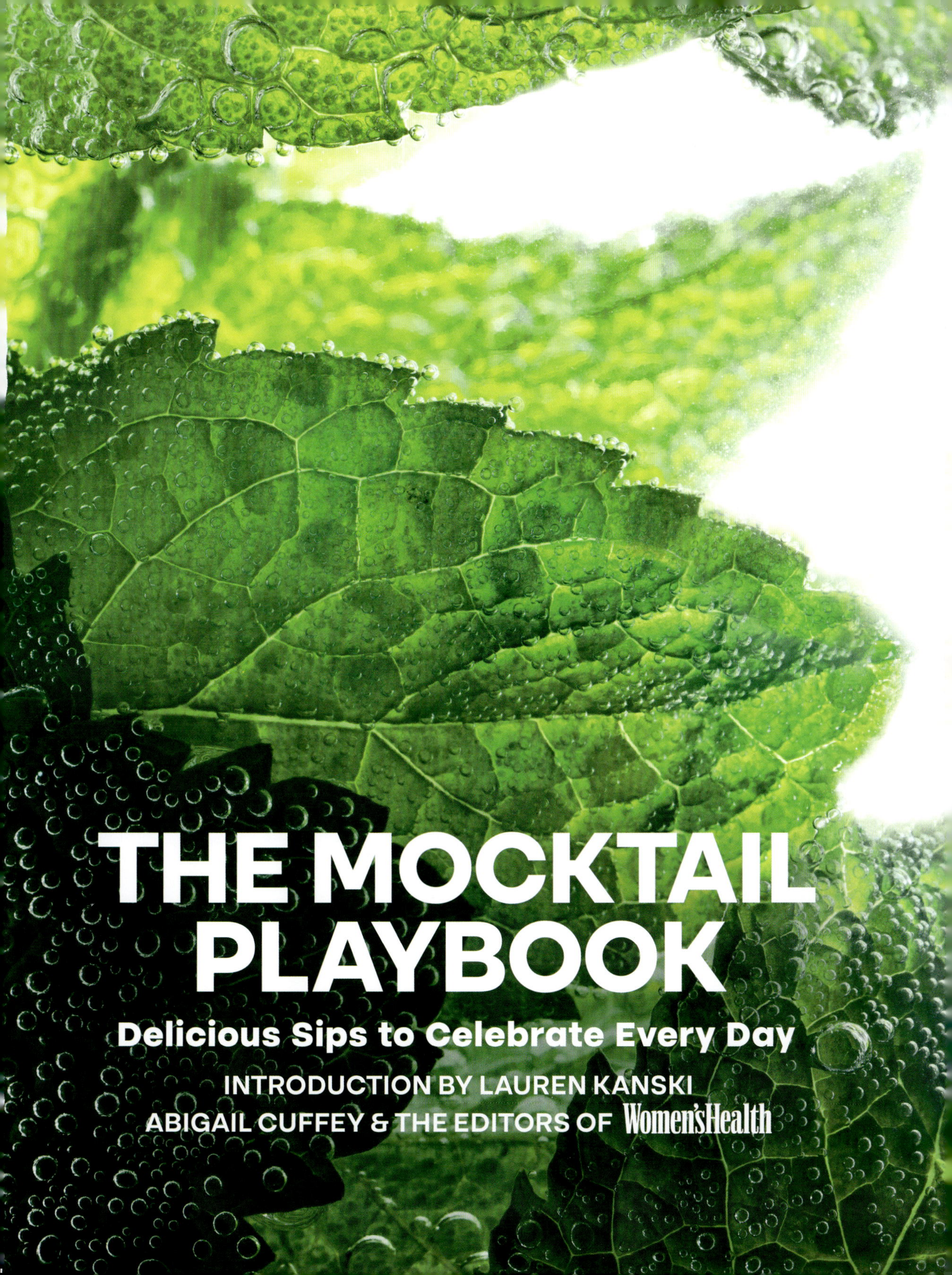
THE MOCKTAIL PLAYBOOK
Delicious Sips to Celebrate Every Day
INTRODUCTION BY LAUREN KANSKI
ABIGAIL CUFFEY & THE EDITORS OF Women'sHealth

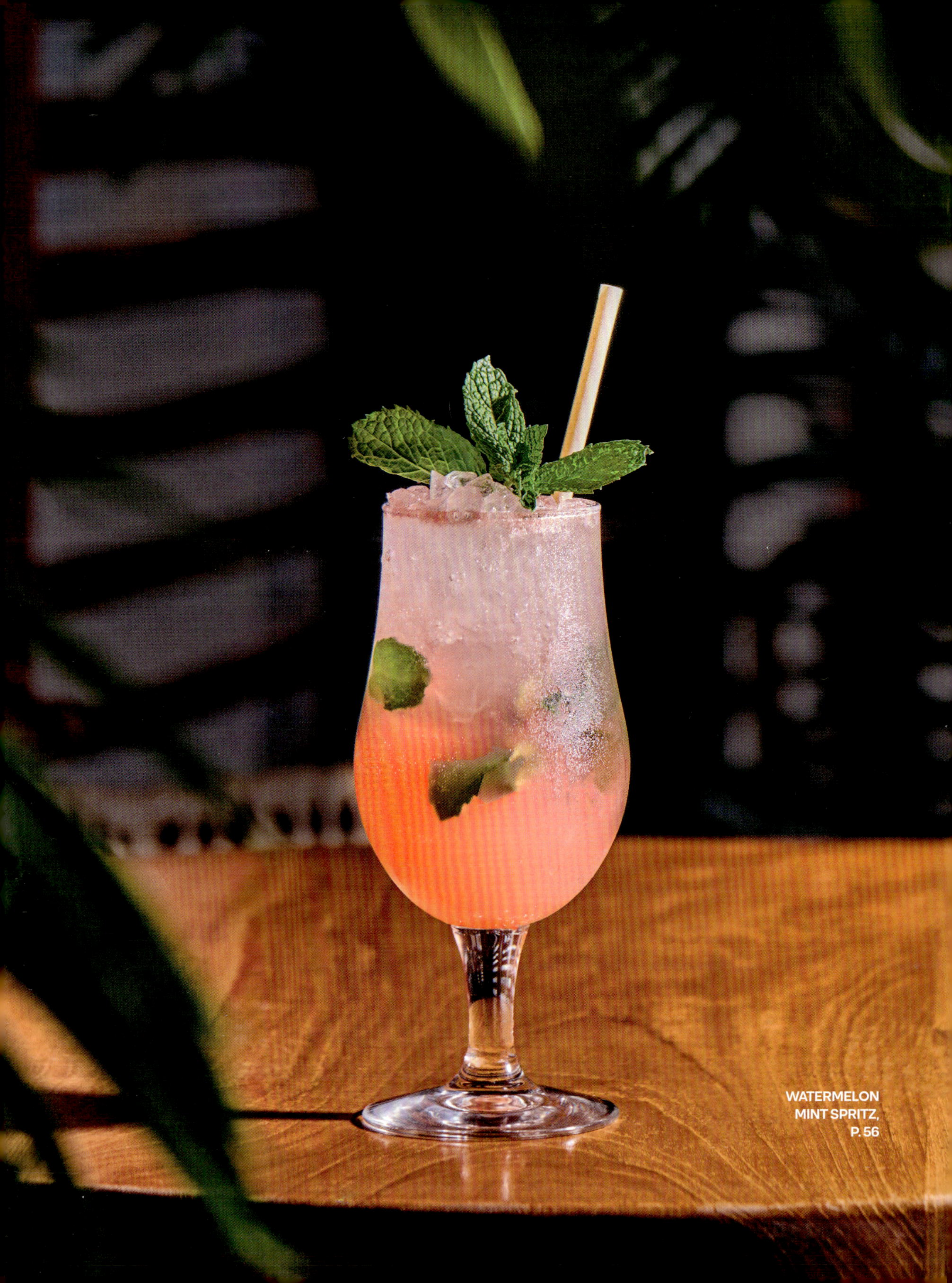

WATERMELON MINT SPRITZ,
P. 56

Contents

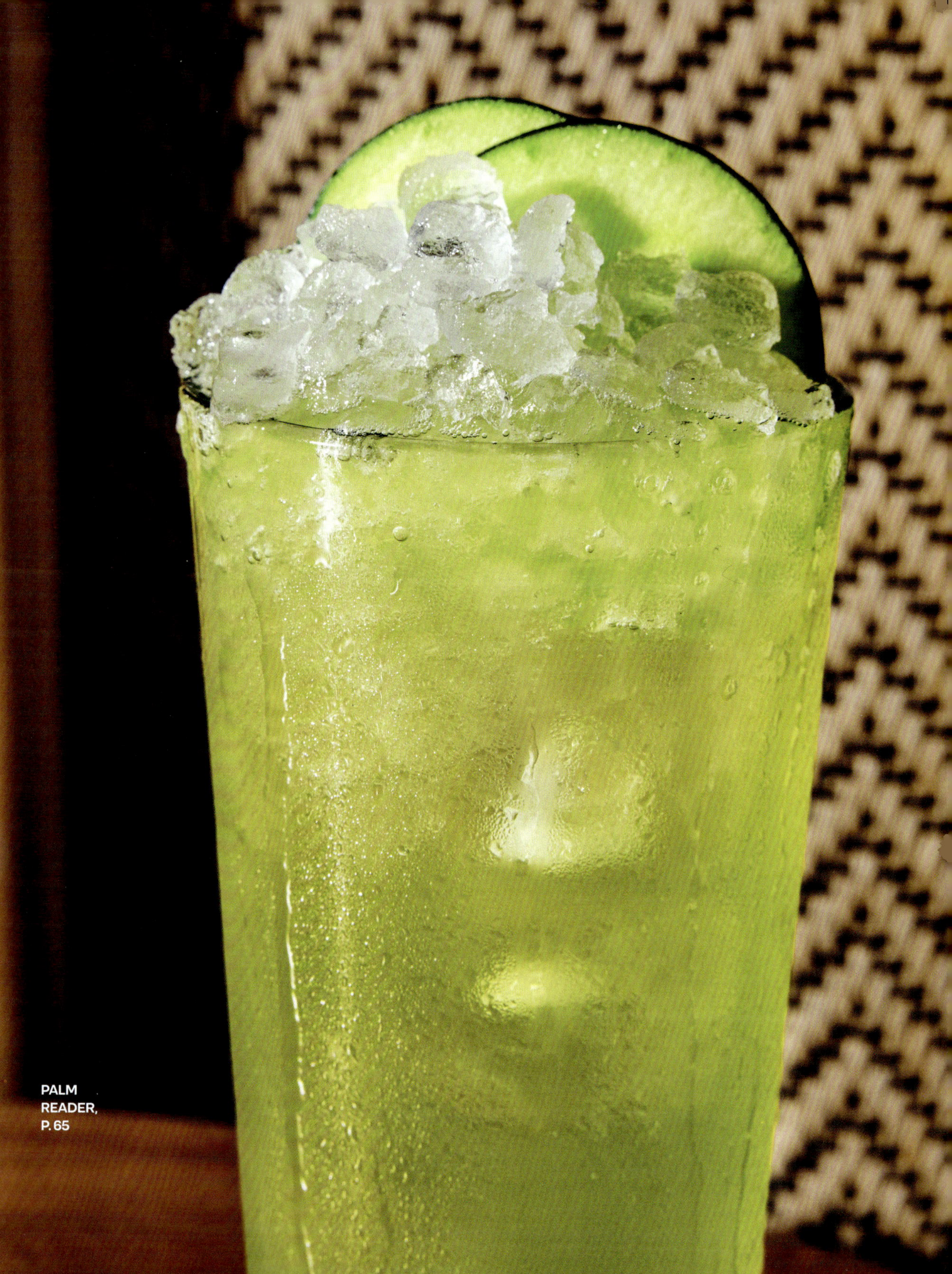

PALM READER, P. 65

A BREAK FROM BOOZE

You know that breakup where nothing awful occurred, but you just knew in your gut that the relationship wasn't right for you anymore? Maybe you even hoped something bad would happen, so it would be easier to walk away?

That was my relationship with alcohol. I didn't have a "problem." No jail time, DUIs, public humiliations, or life-altering consequences. Actually, I have only fond memories from drinking and the fun it brought into my life for over 15 years. That's probably why it took me so long to break up with it.

But I finally did. I cut alcohol cold turkey, about three years ago.

I was just about to turn 30. My husband and I were running the New York City rat race, work was all-consuming and stressful, and our marriage was more like two annoyed roommates living together. Our lives were moving fast—I was gunning it at work, going out after (or decompressing with wine on the couch), and waking early to hit the gym and do it all again. On the weekends, freed from that routine, I drank more to let loose. Things felt, well, blurry. My hangovers kept getting worse. I'd lost the joy in being out late, and I'd regularly experience crippling anxiety after a weekend bender. Still, alcohol remained a crutch.

The wake-up call: My husband and I returned from a 10-day jaunt to Europe, where we had been overindulging (let's be real—binge drinking), and I had a deep gut prompting that I needed a detox. I had never known my life without alcohol in it, and I was curious about who that girl was. I committed to 30 days without alcohol. This challenge would be one of the hardest but most pivotal decisions of my life.

The first week felt easy because it was still new. The second and third weeks were harder because I realized how many of my friendships revolved around trying new restaurants and... drinking. I felt the social pressure more than any internal desire to back out of the bet with myself. This made me question my identity and friendships, but not from a judgmental place.

At the end of the month, I had a spiritual breakthrough. Being sober lifted the fog from my life, which created openness. I reignited faith in my religion. It wasn't until I eliminated alcohol that I entered the space to realize my full potential. My husband and I started to grow toward each other instead of away. I became pregnant with my daughter only two months later. My conversations, memories, and the sheer substance of my life became richer. My friendships evolved; those centered around alcohol fell away, while others grew stronger. I learned to sit with grief and cope with my feelings. I got strong in the gym. These days, I sleep like a baby, so my energy is through the roof, and I recover better. I am now a mom of two, a friend, and a coach, empowering women to make their own realizations along their own journey.

When I cut out "spirits," I finally filled my spirit. If you're feeling the same quiet tug that I did—the nudge that your relationship with alcohol might not be serving you—consider this your invitation. The pages ahead are designed to help—with expert strategies for cutting back, tips for loving your social life without alcohol, success stories, and 50 delicious, simple mocktail recipes to ensure you won't feel deprived in the least.

Whether you decide to take a brief hiatus from alcohol, drink less long term, or cut it out forever, you're about to discover how great life can be when you reassess what's in your glass.

Lauren Kanski, certified personal trainer, *Women's Health* advisory board member

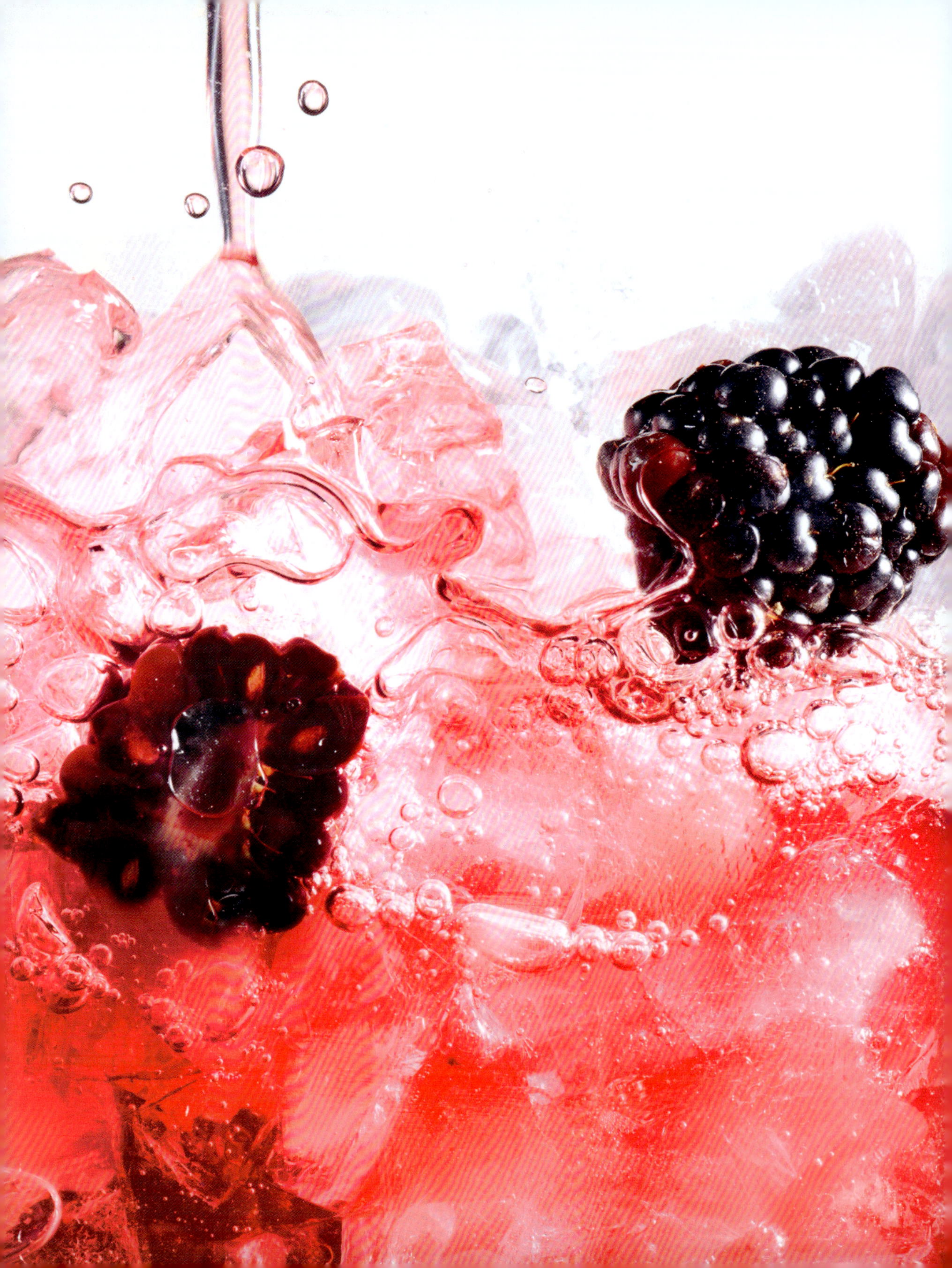

CHAPTER ONE

Drink Less + Live More

» From the condition of your skin to how deeply you sleep, alcohol broadly affects your body and your life. So when you start cutting back, even for a bit, the benefits stack up!

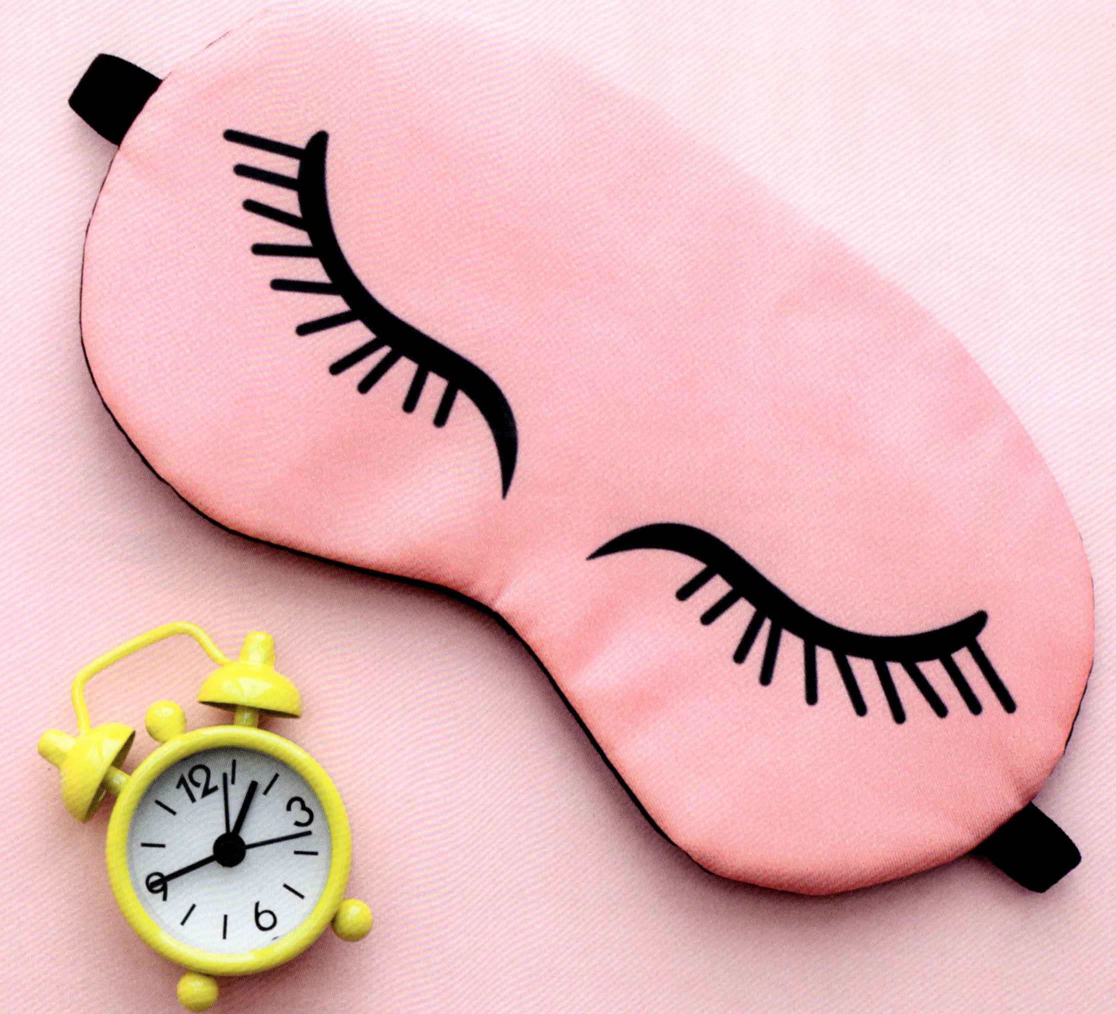

The Health Benefits of Scaling Back

Why a month of drying out could be the reset you need.

Going alcohol-free forever may not seem doable for you. However, there are huge benefits to a hiatus, as those who have tried Dry January or successfully taken an extended break from alcohol at any time can attest. A one-month streak is worth a try, according to Rachel E.K. Freedman, PhD, a licensed psychologist in Bethesda, Maryland.

Even if you don't complete the full streak, stopping for any amount of time is likely to make you feel better. On the other hand, you may appreciate the benefits so much that you keep going way beyond 30 days.

"For some people, for various reasons, the idea of quitting permanently is overwhelming, or they have ideas tied up with what it means to be sober: 'How will I ever have fun again?' Or, 'what will people think?'" says Freedman. "Quitting for one month is seen as doable."

What kind of health advantages is a dry month likely to confer? Plenty, but be patient. You may not notice them within the first month, says Trang M. Vu, MD, an internal medicine physician at UW Medicine in Washington. If you continue limiting your alcohol intake or abstain altogether, you'll notice even more of the benefits.

1. You'll sleep better and have more energy.

"It may sound counterintuitive, since most of us are likely to quickly pass out asleep after a night of drinking more than usual, but too much alcohol screws with your sleep," says Brigitte Zeitlin, RD, CDN, MPH, founder of BZ Nutrition in New York City. After a few drinks, you're less able to reach deep sleep, which helps your body de-stress, repair, and replenish itself for the next day, she says.

When you ditch the alcohol, however, you won't have those restless nights. "Practicing a sober month will help you sleep and feel rested and energized in the mornings," says Zeitlin.

2. Your skin could clear up.

Alcohol is a diuretic, which means it can make you go to the bathroom more frequently—and ultimately leave you dehydrated, says Zeitlin. That dehydration can take a serious toll on your skin. "By ditching the alcohol and upping your

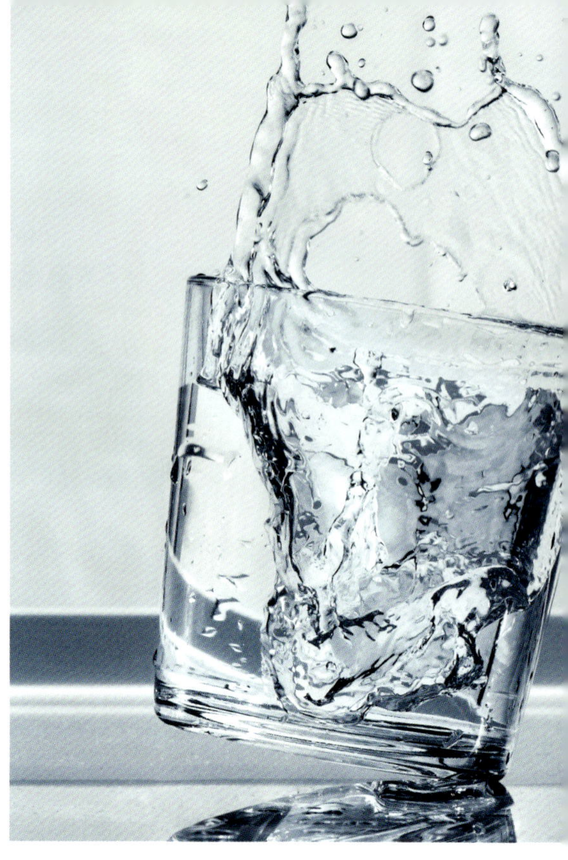

HOW DRY JANUARY BEGAN

Dry January was launched in England in 2013 by the nonprofit Alcohol Change UK to raise awareness and funds for alcohol abuse treatment. The concept quickly caught on.

water intake, it's a win-win for your hydration status and will leave your skin feeling healthier and looking more radiant," Zeitlin says.

Plus, the high sugar content in alcoholic beverages may trigger your body to produce the hormone IGF-1, which can cause an overproduction of oil in your skin (hi, pimples!). Pair this with spiking blood sugar levels that promote inflammation, and you've got yourself a recipe for acne. So, losing the booze can potentially improve acne for those who have it.

3. You may lose weight.

Dropping pounds when you go sober is pretty standard, says Zeitlin—in fact, if you were to make zero other changes to your diet except for cutting alcohol, you'd still probably lose weight.

"One alcoholic drink is typically 150 to 200 calories, which can really add up," Zeitlin says. "Additionally, when we drink a lot we tend to eat more than we realize, so cutting back on the alcohol will likely help you to cut down on some of the mindless overeating that usually happens after the third round of cocktails."

As a bonus, you may find that you are less bloated or puffy without those nights of drinking too much, which in turn will make you feel better in your body, Zeitlin says.

4. Your immune system could get stronger.

Drinking a lot can suppress your immune function, which can make you more vulnerable to the pathogens that cause the cold and flu, says Keri Peterson, MD, a *Women's Health* advisory board member. In addition, frequent drinking can cause inflammation throughout the body. All of this means that taking a break from booze could help you better fight off seasonal illnesses.

5. You may feel less anxious.

The day after drinking, you may have the nausea and headache that come with a hangover. But you may also experience "hangxiety," or anxious feelings, Dr. Peterson says. If you stay away from booze for a month, you'll be hangover- and hangxiety-free, enjoying more peaceful nights and less worrisome mornings, according to Dr. Peterson.

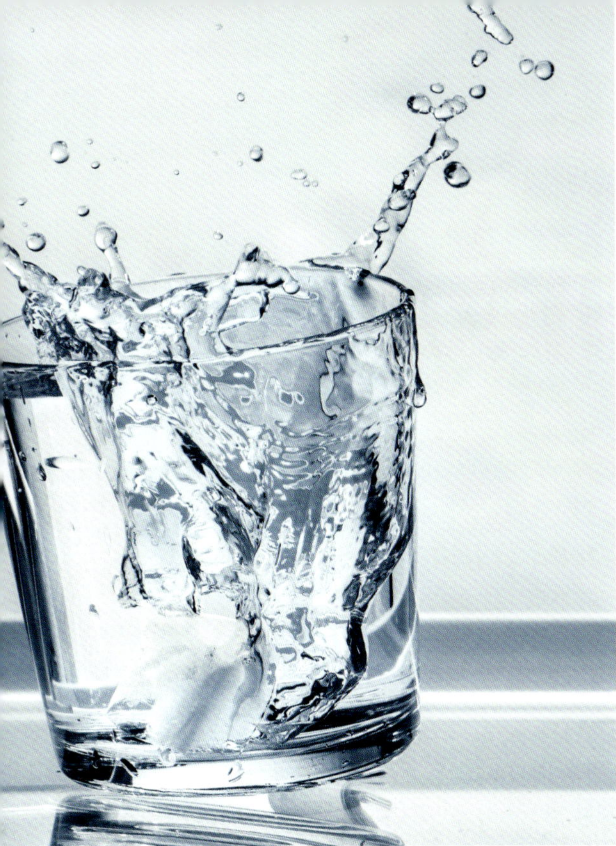

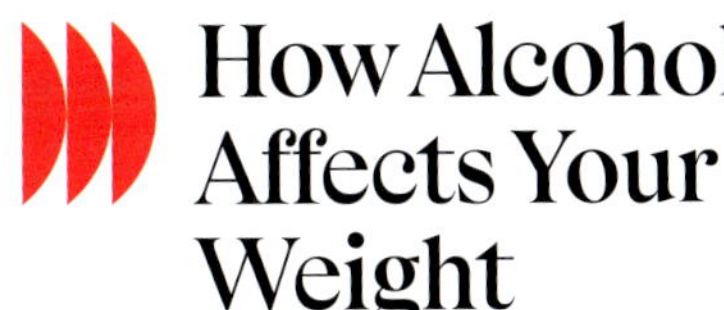

How Alcohol Affects Your Weight

The role drinking plays in your diet can impact your weight in some surprising ways. Alcohol lowers your inhibitions and makes it harder to focus during meals, which can lead to overeating or choosing foods you otherwise wouldn't, says Marissa Karp, RD, the founder of MPM Nutrition.

Additionally, alcohol can cause your blood sugar to drop, increasing hunger and leading to snacking, according to Tanya Mezher, RD, a lead functional practitioner at Malla.

Even hangovers can interfere with healthy eating and exercise. "If we wake up hungover, we are more likely to skip our normal workout class or grocery shopping and, instead, order [takeout] and not move," adds Karp. If and when you do decide to drink, it's best to keep your beverages light, low-sugar, and low-calorie.

Booze can also exacerbate how you react to stress, says Molly Kimball, RD, founder of the Ochsner Eat Fit initiative in New Orleans. Something that might elicit a 3 on a 1-to-10 stress scale when sober could reach an 8 after drinking, she explains. "Most people find they handle stressful situations better without alcohol."

6. You'll have fewer headaches.

Another benefit of not drinking? Fewer headaches, says Dr. Peterson. These are usually brought on by the dehydration that happens when you drink. They're also a classic hangover symptom that you won't have to worry about during your dry month.

7. Your overall health will improve.

As your body adjusts to a lack of alcohol, your blood pressure will likely lower and your liver will heal from any effects of heavy or binge drinking, says Dr. Peterson.

If you're engaged in binge drinking (for women, four or more drinks in two hours) or heavy drinking (eight or more drinks in one week), you may want to consult your doctor before abruptly quitting, says Trang M. Vu, MD, a physician at UW Medicine in Washington. In some cases, "Stopping can lead to withdrawal [symptoms]." Your doctor can help you determine how best to stop drinking based on your habits.

Rethinking Drinking

Teenagers and 20-somethings are far less interested in alcohol than those who came before them. Learn what's driving the appeal of abstinence.

Drinking was once sewn into the experience of one's 20s: alcohol-fueled nights on the town, hazy after-work happy hours, and raucous Saturday-morning bottomless brunches were ubiquitous. But today's 20-somethings are rewriting that script.

"Among Gen Z [those born between 1997 and 2012], the proportion of people who choose not to drink is increasing by about half a percentage point annually," says Ziming Xuan, a social epidemiologist and professor of community health sciences at Boston University. According to a 2020 study in *JAMA Pediatrics*, 28 percent of college students in 2018 reported abstaining from alcohol; only 20 percent did so in 2002. A larger proportion of people choose not to drink, "and those who choose to drink tend to drink less," Xuan says.

What's driving the trend? "The effect alcohol has on physical health and mental health is evident," says Hilary Sheinbaum, author of *Going Dry*. For starters, there's a greater awareness of alcohol's role in the development of cancer and other diseases. But its impact on emotional health is also better appreciated now.

Nearly two-thirds of British consumers between the ages of 18 and 24 are worried about the emotional impact of alcohol, according to a Mintel survey from 2023. Junia Lebek, a graduate student and "retired party girl," says she stopped drinking in her junior year of college. "My mental health got so bad that [alcohol was] the only coping mechanism," she says. Sober for more than five years, she's never felt better.

Writer Mary Honkus began to abstain after "I noticed that anytime that I would drink, my hangovers weren't just physical," she says. "I would find myself in depressive states that would last for weeks. And I wasn't the kind of person who drank every day; I was a social drinker."

If Gen X grew up thinking drinking was cool, their kids see it otherwise: More than half of Gen Zers worry about how too much drinking might make them look, according to research from the British agencies Red Brick Road and Opinium. "I'm not super interested in being out of control," says Nat Segebre, a photographer.

Jade Corona, a publicist, concurs: "As someone who likes to be in control, I felt like [alcohol] would take me out of control. I just didn't think it was cool."

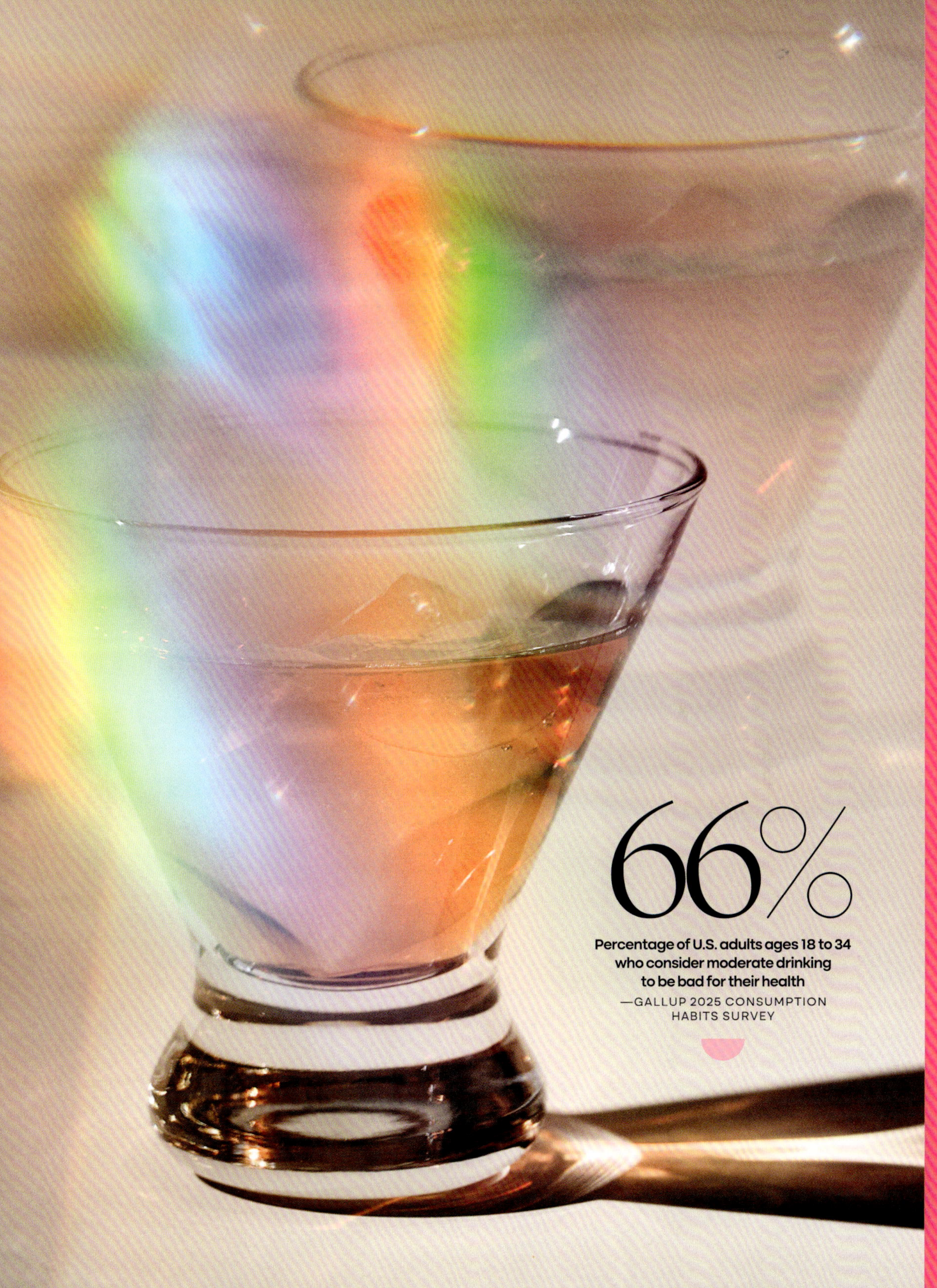

66%

Percentage of U.S. adults ages 18 to 34 who consider moderate drinking to be bad for their health

—GALLUP 2025 CONSUMPTION HABITS SURVEY

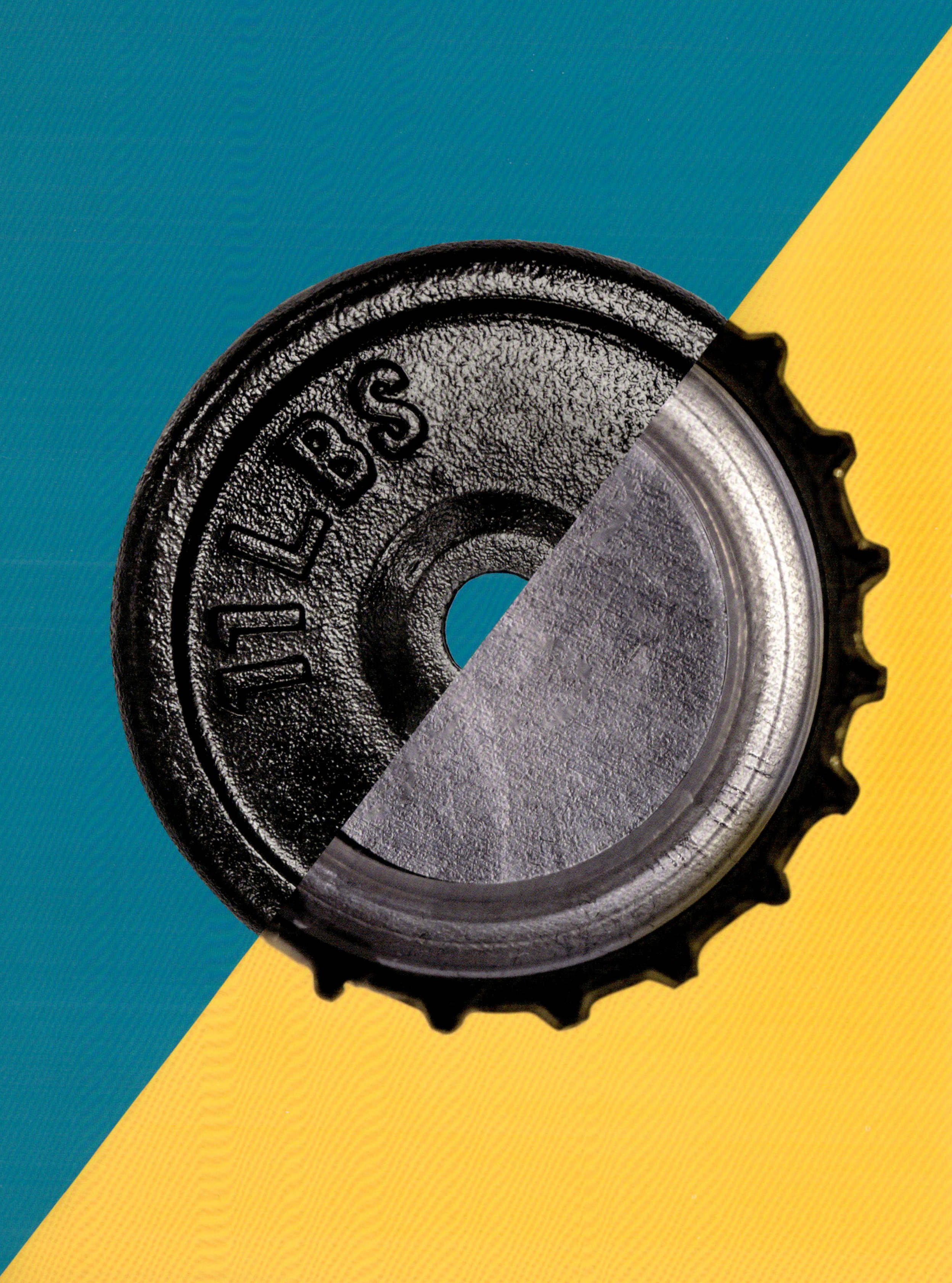
11 LBS

How Alcohol Impacts Your Workout

Abstaining can be a boon not just for your gym attendance but for your performance and recovery, too. Try these tactics.

Drinking and workouts tend to have an inverse relationship, as anyone who's flaked on gym class after going hard the night before knows. Could scaling back your intake improve the quality of your exercise? It won't hurt.

Cutting back could support your all-around wellness habits, which could improve your workout performance, says Katie Witkiewitz, PhD, director of the University of New Mexico's Center on Alcohol, Substance Use, and Addictions. "Any reduction in drinking is beneficial, as it may help you be more active or competitive because you'll have better sleep, energy, and general physical function."

What exactly does a bev here and there do to your performance? It depends on factors such as age, gender, body mass, and other variables. Generally speaking, when you drink, your body is busy processing that alcohol, hindering muscle repair and hydration—components of recovery that allow you to adapt to the stress of training and to continue exercising.

Also, the more you drink, the more you'll urinate, which impedes the hydration process. Alcohol, too, may inhibit the uptake of certain nutrients and protein synthesis, which stunts muscle repair, and it can reduce production of hormones that help grow muscles, research shows. While you may fall asleep faster after a cocktail, the overall quality of your sleep —the most critical aspect of recovery for athletes—is diminished. Imbibing spurs the liver to metabolize alcohol during the night; as the blood alcohol level decreases, you're more likely to have sleep disruptions.

Ultimately, while science doesn't say for certain that quitting drinking will help you run faster or lift heavier, it's widely accepted that not drinking—for a day, a week, a year, or forever—is likely to positively impact performance

Strike a Balance

For women considering a cutback, Witkiewitz encourages first assessing your drinking habits by keeping a diary or using one of the many apps that allow you to track your consumption. Sarah MacKay Robinson uses a free app called I Am Sober, which lets you list your reasons for omitting alcohol. When you log in to see how many days you've gone without a drink, you're reminded of your "why." Looking ahead can also be inspirational. Robinson uses an upcoming fitness event as a motivation to stay dry. "I would post the date of the race to have that front and center," she says.

After you track your drinks for a month or so, identify the sips you could reasonably cut out. Some people choose not to have alcohol on weekdays, for example, or commit to one glass of wine with dinner instead of two. Planning ahead lets you see where you intend to imbibe. If you're tracking total drinks per week and know an event is coming up where you'll want to indulge, you can adjust your consumption for the rest of the week accordingly.

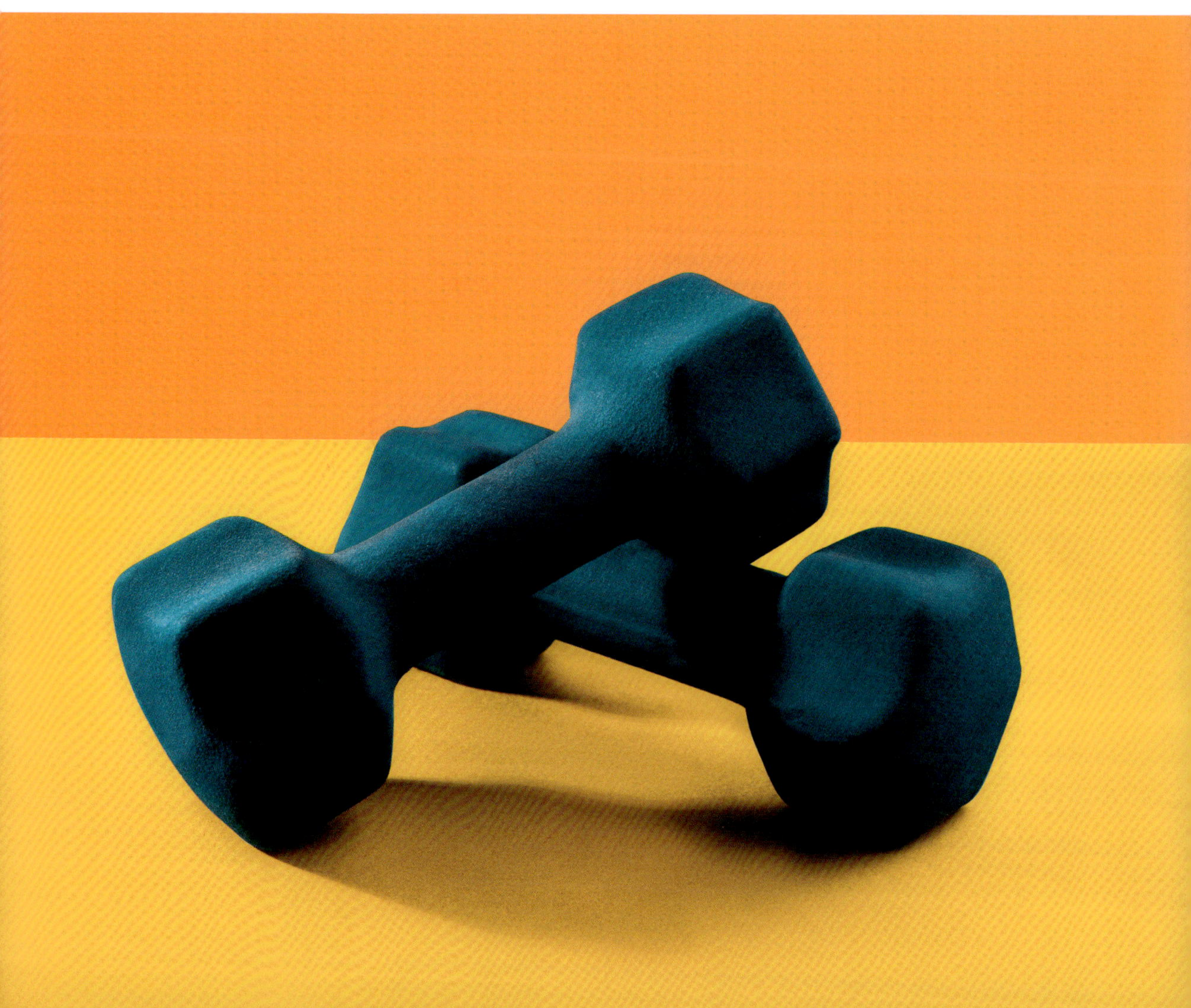

Rachel Gersten, a therapist in New York who cut out alcohol to manage an inflammatory autoimmune disease, encourages the sober curious to try a dry period and see what happens. She believes most people would be surprised by how much alcohol pops up in their life and how it requires intention to adjust their ingrained drinking rituals. "Try to gather information about yourself," Gersten says. That information can be valuable both in and out of the gym.

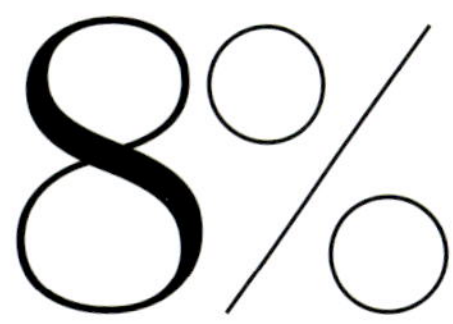

The average decline in next-day recovery after drinking alcohol the day before. Consuming alcohol had the single greatest negative impact on next-day recovery of all the trackable metrics on the WHOOP health app.

Cutting Back Fueled Their Fitness!

• **When Stevie Lyn Smith, RD,** lived in Washington, DC, a few years ago, she trained for Ironman triathlons—and partook in the heavy happy hour culture. She'd have a few cocktails and get up the next day to train, even when she was hung over. Then a move to Buffalo coincided with the onset of the pandemic, which tabled socializing. It didn't take long for her to notice how much better she felt without alcohol.

She could wake up on Sunday mornings and not want to stay in bed all day. The data backed up what she felt, too—her sports watch tracked stats such as heart rate variability (or HRV, the variation in time between each beat), a measure that increased the less she drank, indicating greater fitness and better recovery. (The number usually drops if you're sick, tired, stressed, or otherwise struggling.) "Because of my Ironman background, I live and die by heart rate training. When I was drinking, my heart rate was higher, and I'd just drag in workouts," says Smith, who also counsels other athletes on fueling their active lives.

Smith hasn't cut out all alcohol, but she limits it considerably these days, usually to when she's going to a restaurant that has a well-made cocktail or to a hard seltzer at a baseball game with her mom. "It's a very intentional choice," she says. "I often go months without a drink."

Many of Smith's nutrition clients inquire about cutting down while they're training for an endurance event. Usually, they have a hunch about what she's going to say. "Most people come to me already knowing that drinking is probably not the best choice for their goal and what they're looking to do," she says. When they get honest with her about alcohol, Smith says, "They tend to at least adjust their behaviors around it because they start to recognize that it's detrimental."

• **Whenever Lindsay Riess** begins another 12-week training cycle in which she'll run up to 70 miles per week to hit a personal record in a marathon, she cuts out alcohol. She can't tell if the decision has had any obvious effect on her results, but the habit makes her feel healthier overall. Her one exception? The runner, who lives in Arizona, still likes to have one anticipatory drink the night before a marathon. "It takes that anxiety piece down for me, so that's my little contradiction," she says.

• **Sarah MacKay Robinson** has gone without a drink for more than two years and experienced her best training and fastest marathon after three months completely dry (coincidence or not). She admits only one regret about her decision to eliminate alcohol: "I wish I did it sooner, when I was at my peak fitness, because I would've crushed."

Alcohol and Menopause

Many women are sensitive to even a drink or two at this stage of life. Reducing your intake can ease this transition.

You knew that hot flashes were part of the deal, but perimenopause and menopause can also affect how your body responds to drinking. It's not your imagination: These life stages amplify the alcohol's negative impact.

"Declining estrogen at menopause can impact alcohol metabolism," says Juliana (Jewel) Kling, MD, chair of Women's Health Internal Medicine at Mayo Clinic Alix School of Medicine, Arizona campus. "Alcohol can also increase the risk of osteoporosis, breast cancer, and heart disease, all diagnoses that women are at higher risk of post-menopause." Drinking can also worsen menopause symptoms, such as hot flashes, she adds.

Scaling back alcohol (along with healthy eating and exercise) during this time of your life can improve a slew of unpleasant symptoms and also lessen your risk of chronic disease, says Dr. Kling.

Why Alcohol Is Detrimental

First, know this: "Women [of any age] are more susceptible than men to the adverse effects of alcohol because there [are fewer] enzymes in the stomach to neutralize it," says Deborah Gomez Kwolek, MD, an assistant professor of medicine at Harvard Medical School and the founding lead of the Mass General Women's Health and Sex and Gender Medicine Program. From the stomach, it floods the liver, putting the organ into overdrive. During menopause, alcohol's impact on your liver—and entire metabolic system—compounds, which could up your risk for fatty liver, high cholesterol, and diabetes.

Meno-Belly, Insomnia, and More

If you're concerned about "meno belly"—excess fat stored in the waist due to waning estrogen—know that alcohol can contribute to that bloat. Drinking also disrupts sleep, can worsen hot flashes, and even moderate drinking is considered a significant risk factor for breast cancer. "You have to realize that [drinking] really is not doing your body a favor," Dr. Kwolek says.

Paring Back for an Easier "Pause"

"If you cut back, you're going to feel so much better," Dr. Kwolek says. You'll likely feel more energized since you'll sleep better, she says. On the health front, by removing alcohol, you help your liver detoxify and reduce your disease risk. You may also lose weight, Dr. Kling adds.

All of your health-conscious changes go hand in hand, Dr. Kwolek says. "I talk to my patients about lifestyle medicine: exercise, nutrition, sleep, stress reduction, and avoiding toxins (e.g., alcohol) are five big pillars of that."

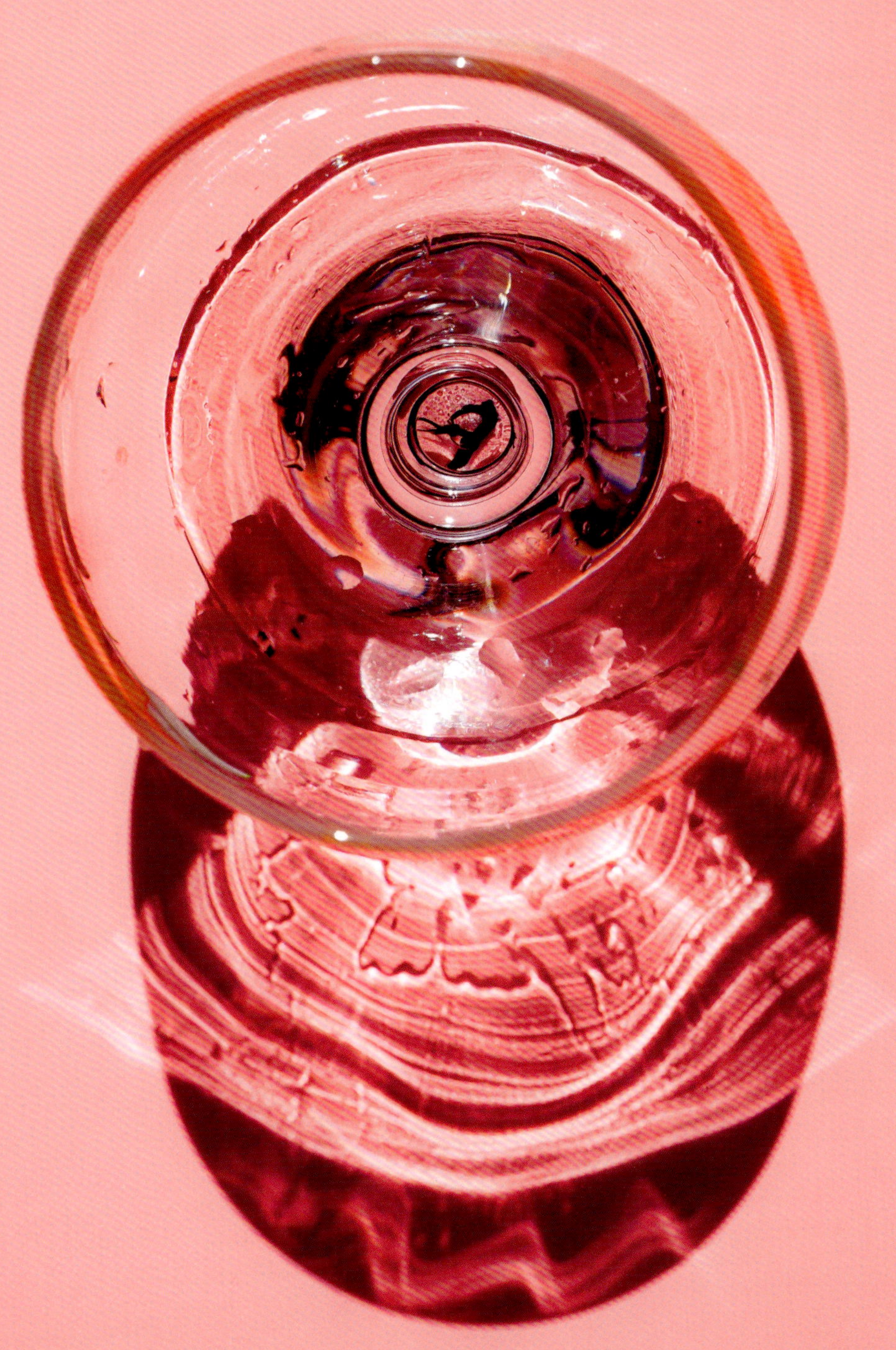

Why Go Dry?

Until recently, social drinking was thought of as relatively harmless. Its effect on our health is now clearer.

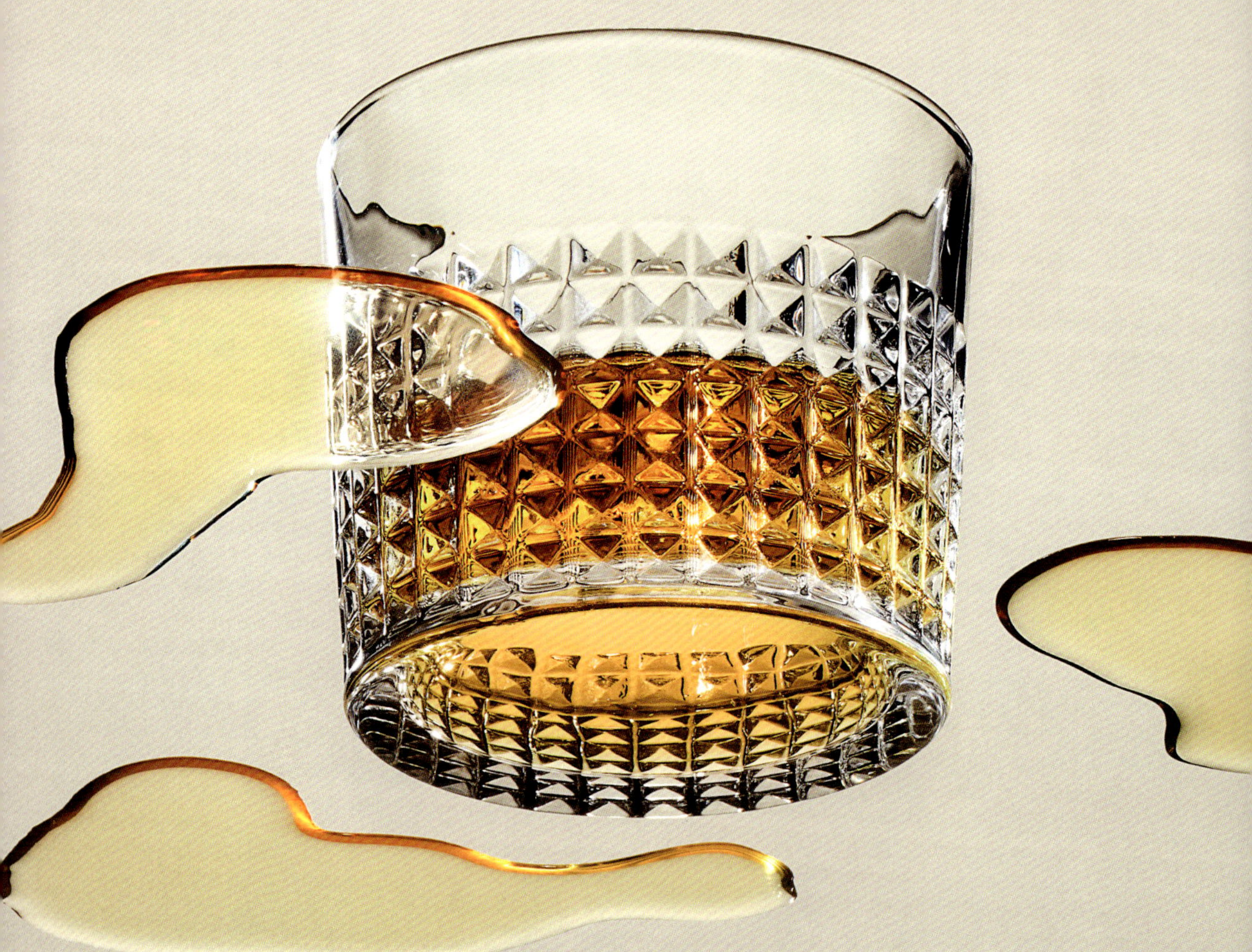

Alcohol has held a special, complicated spot in our culture for ages: It's synonymous with celebrating, a reliable social lubricant, a time-honored way to shrug off the day's stresses. Yet mounting research shows that drinking also plays a role in disease and mental decline. Is it time to adjust our habits to keep pace with the latest science?

For decades, scientists have known that drinking is linked to serious health risks, including several cancers. The World Health Organization (WHO) first declared alcohol a known carcinogen back in 1987. Yet even today, many people are in the dark regarding the damage alcohol can do. Sales have remained strong—in 2024, the alcohol market declined only slightly. However, the drumbeat about the dangers of drinking has grown louder.

In 2023, public health leaders at the WHO declared that no amount of alcohol consumption is safe. Research has shown that it can play a role in more than 200 types of disease and health issues, from heart disease and cancer to dementia and depression. Drinking remains a major part of modern culture, family traditions, and our Friday night plans. Yet a growing number of people are abstaining. Only 54 percent of Americans drink, the lowest since Gallup began tracking drinking trends in 1939.

Even moderate drinking—one drink or fewer a day for women, per the CDC—can carry long-term health risks, although the less you drink, the less likely you are to experience serious repercussions. So do we need to give it up?

The Health Halo Effect

Part of what makes the news of alcohol's health risks confusing is that we were once told the opposite. In the 1990s, a wave of studies suggested that drinking—especially red wine—might protect against heart disease. The idea gained traction in 1991, when a *60 Minutes* segment shared a French researcher's suggestion that consuming alcohol offered a protective effect against heart disease. The segment explored the "French Paradox" (the perception that despite eating high-fat diets, French people had low rates of heart disease), which the researcher suggested had to do with eating cheese rather than drinking milk, and consuming alcohol.

40%

Share of American drinkers polled who hadn't imbibed in more than a week. This is the highest percentage since 2000.

—GALLUP 2025 CONSUMPTION HABITS SURVEY

Over the years, several dozen studies came to similar findings: that people who consumed one or two drinks a day had a 25 percent lower risk of cardiovascular disease or coronary disease mortality. Data suggested that those abstaining from alcohol had a higher risk of health issues, says James Morris, who researches alcohol and stigma at London South Bank University. When small studies suggested that the antioxidant compound resveratrol, found in red wine, could inhibit the formation of blood clots and break down fats, it seemed to solidify the link between alcohol and good health.

Early on, researchers identified issues with how these studies were constructed, but their concerns were overshadowed by the volume of research that funding from the alcohol industry enabled, according to David Nutt, a professor of neuropsychopharmacology at Imperial College London. "The drinks industry has been phenomenally clear at promoting the possible

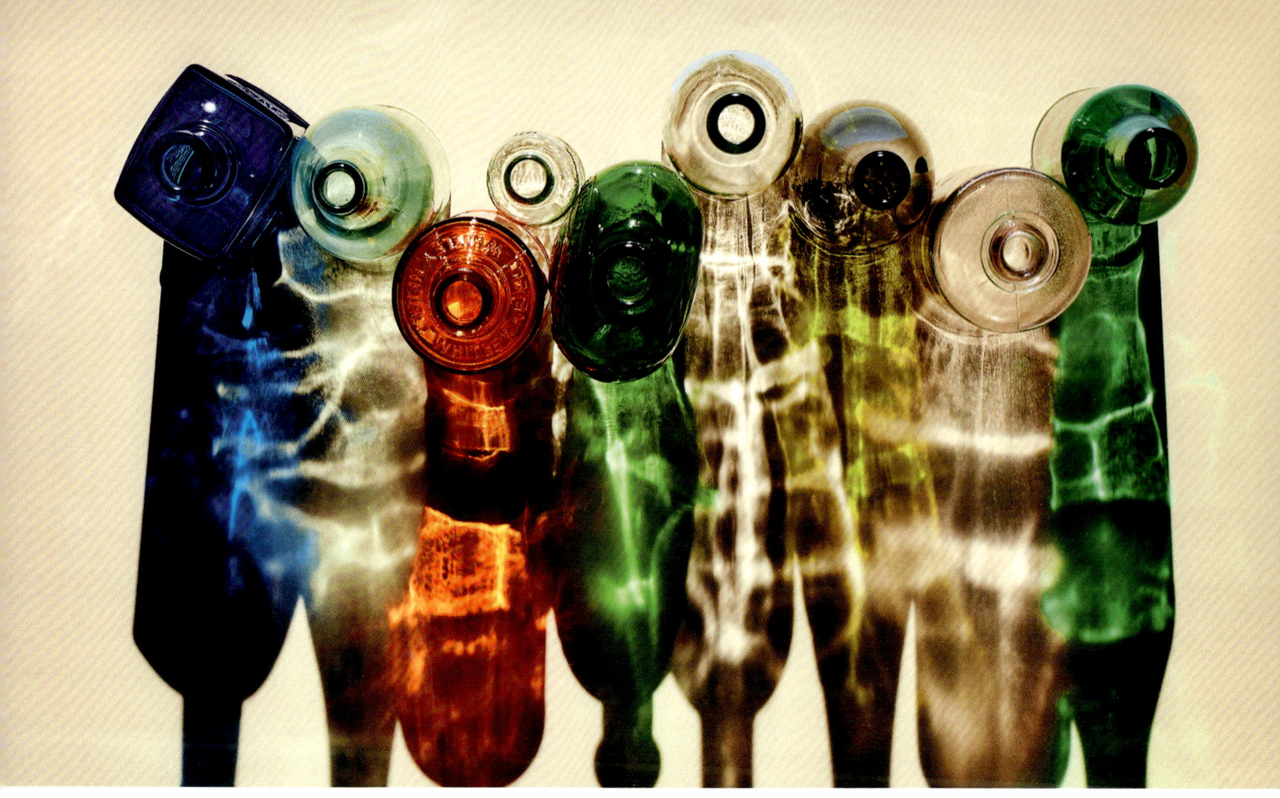

benefits of alcohol, or undermining people's criticism of the benefits," he says.

It makes sense that we'd lean into any good news about a beverage that has helped prop up most of our civilizations, says Nutt. Low-alcohol beers likely provided essential calories and nutrients in early Europe and Africa, and wine's ritual importance in multiple major religions stretches far back. "It was beer that brought humans together, not bread," Nutt says.

The Studies' Shortcomings

It took scientists until the 2010s to identify the flaws in these studies. As Nutt explains, researchers weren't accounting for why the non-drinkers were abstaining. When recruiting nondrinking participants, they didn't ask those people if they'd ever been drinkers, or why they didn't currently drink. Many nondrinkers had stopped due to illness or substance abuse, which skewed the results. What's more, those moderate drinkers tended to have more money, more education, and better access to health care, other socioeconomic factors that protect against disease. The great French Paradox, according to Nutt, is simply "an artifact of wealth, lots of olive oil, and vitamin D."

In extensive analyses of newer studies, in which the nondrinkers are lifetime abstainers, the data trend tying alcohol to lower mortality tends to disappear. "When they filter out poor-quality studies from those analyses, you just see more drinking, more risk," says Morris.

Regarding research on red wine and resveratrol, the dose of resveratrol required to produce even a small heart-healthy effect is so large that wine alone is insufficient. Studies linking resveratrol to heart health typically were based on users taking at least 100 milligrams per day, in supplement form. A 5-ounce glass of red wine contains just 1 to 2 milligrams of resveratrol, which means you'd need to drink upward of 50 glasses of wine a day—a prescription no doctor is writing.

How Alcohol Impacts Health

The truth is, alcohol can affect nearly every system in the body. The alcohol-cancer connection is particularly concerning. While a whole constellation of personal risk factors and behaviors contributes to cancer development, alcohol is among them. Alcohol's most abundant metabolite (a substance produced when your body breaks it down), acetaldehyde, is a carcinogen. It damages DNA and disrupts the body's repair processes, and it's linked to colorectal, esophageal, and other types of cancer. Alcohol also alters the mouth's microbiome, contributing to oral cancers.

Alcohol's correlation with breast cancer is far more significant than for other types, according to Morris. A meta-analysis back in 2002 found that women who consumed two alcoholic drinks per day had a 14 percent higher lifetime risk for breast cancer than those who didn't. Globally, alcohol is believed to be responsible for roughly 100,000 breast cancer cases each year. Alcohol contributes to one in every six breast cancer cases, according to former U.S. Surgeon General Vivek Murthy, MD.

And yet, two-thirds of American respondents in a 2019 health survey were unaware of alcohol's role in cancer. Even those in the know may brush away these stats by leaning into "cancer fatalism"—the idea that "everything causes cancer, so there's nothing you can do to prevent it," says Kara Wiseman, PhD, an epidemiologist at the University of Virginia School of Medicine. That outlook can keep you from making informed health decisions, including whether and how much to drink.

Evidence of drinking's impact on brain health can also be difficult to grapple with, says Anya Topiwala, MD, a psychiatrist at the University of Oxford—particularly because experts are still trying to determine how alcohol's impacts play out on an individual level. Scientists do know that excessive alcohol consumption can affect the neurons that make up the brain and central nervous system. In Dr. Topiwala's own work, she found that drinking more than four to eight standard U.S. drinks a week may accelerate brain aging. Just an extra 1.71 drinks (or roughly 24 grams of ethanol) weekly is "equivalent to an extra year of aging on the brain."

–11%

Drop in the percentage of women who drink, from 62% in 2023 to 51% in 2025

—2025 GALLUP CONSUMPTION HABITS SURVEY

Where to Go From Here

The truth is, no amount of alcohol can be considered good for you. The WHO stated in 2023 that there's no level of alcohol consumption that does not affect your health in some way, and the more you drink, the more harmful it is. But this isn't all doom and gloom. Looked at more positively, cutting back—by dropping drinking during the workweek, stopping at one or two on Saturday night, taking a 30-day hiatus, or stirring up some delicious spirit-free alternatives to the hard stuff (plenty of those coming up!)—can only be beneficial. Giving up alcohol completely and forever may be a wise health move, depending on how much you drink now and whether you have trouble moderating. But being more mindful about how, why, and when you drink brings a boatload of benefits, too. By picking up this book, you've already taken the first step. Enjoy!

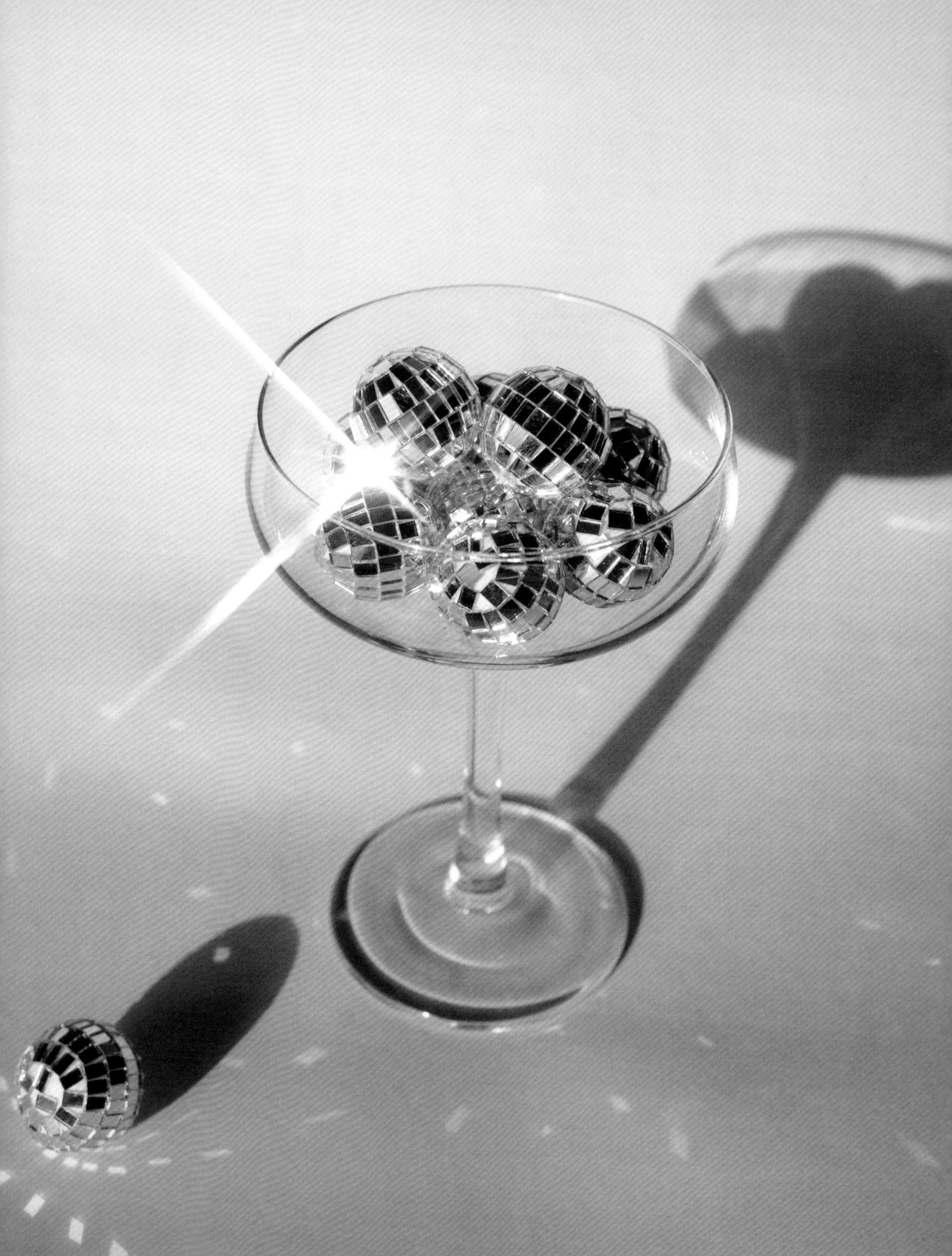

Love Your Social Life Without Alcohol

Keep the friends, the parties, and all the fun—no booze necessary.

If you're exploring what drinking less looks like for you—you're in good company: More people are reevaluating the role that alcohol plays in their lives. Still, it's not always easy, especially when drinking is front and center in so many social settings.

"It's hard to go anywhere without someone offering you a drink," says Leah Young, LCPC, clinical manager for Eating Recovery Center and for Pathlight Mood & Anxiety Centers. Even if you don't struggle with alcohol addiction, reducing your alcohol intake can be difficult.

Alcohol shows up everywhere. It's at happy hours, company events, birthday parties, sports games, funerals, you name it. "It's become almost the main character in social situations," says Hilary Sheinbaum, author of *The Dry Challenge: How to Lose the Booze for Dry January, Sober October, and Any Other Alcohol-Free Month.* "Alcohol has permeated both happy moments and celebrations and sad ones when people are grieving and everything in between." With so many social rituals tied to alcohol, stepping back can feel like falling out of step.

Blame thousands of years of tradition, as well as media messaging and marketing. Alcohol has played a major role in how we bond. It gives us a reason to meet up, and it soothes social awkwardness when we do. So trying to cut back comes with logistical questions. Can you still go to the bar with friends? And how do you explain your choice without people making it a big deal?

Because drinking is so normalized, choosing not to drink can raise questions. You can expect some people to be curious, says Young. Others might seem uncomfortable or disappointed.

But those reactions can be thought of as more of a "them thing, and less of a you thing," says Shani Gardner, LCSW, founder of Soulful Grace Therapy. Approach those moments with compassion, don't take it personally, she says.

At the same time, you might interpret neutral reactions as judgment. "We fill in the gaps in our head with what we think other people are thinking," says Hayley Treloar Padovano, PhD, an associate professor of behavioral and social sciences at the Center for Alcohol and Addiction Studies at Brown University School of Public Health. "A lot of times those things aren't true."

Drinking less (or not at all) doesn't need to dull your social spark. "You're still going to be fun. You're still going to be as engaged—if not more engaged—in the conversation," says Sheinbaum. "It's just that you're holding something different in your hands." Try these tactics for being out and about without alcohol.

1. Practice turning down alcohol in advance.

If you're heading to an event where you'll likely be offered a drink, plan what you'll say. You don't owe anyone an explanation, but coming up with something short and sweet beforehand can help you feel confident. "You can have one [line] ready to go for everybody, or you can tailor it depending on your relationship with the person," says Young. But so you don't freeze and fumble, "it's important to practice it."

You can stick to something simple, like, "Thanks, but I have a huge day at work tomorrow," or "Actually, what I'm really craving right now is a Diet Coke." Or, if you feel like sharing, "I'm cutting back to see if it helps my energy or focus." You might even find that others have the same goal.

But how you say it matters. Confidence is key, says Young. Don't be afraid to be firm if you need to be, adds Sheinbaum. And don't be surprised if friends turn out to have a similar goal.

2. Delay your first drink by 30 minutes.

Ordering a drink as soon as you arrive is a reflex. Give yourself a half hour to settle in before deciding if you really want one. This mini-experiment can help you learn to tolerate social discomfort without immediately reaching for a drink. Your anxiety may start to fade on its own. "Our anxiety just can't keep going up forever," says Padovano. With practice, you build the muscle to navigate social spaces without leaning on alcohol. Once the 30 minutes are up, go ahead and order a drink, if you still want it. Or you might decide to skip it entirely.

3. Take the lead when ordering or making plans.

Ever notice how one person's order can influence the whole table? The first person to order gets an espresso martini, and then suddenly everyone else at the table orders one, too. Drinking is often about sharing an experience, says Sheinbaum. That experience

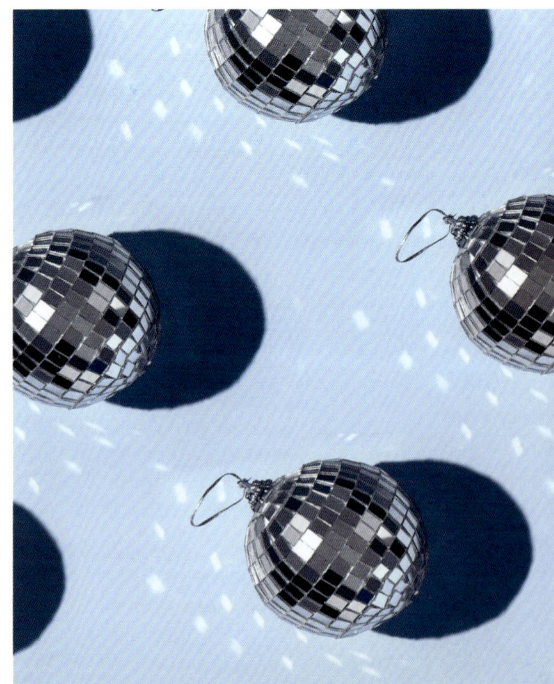

doesn't need to involve alcohol. Be the one to set the tone by ordering a mocktail or the house-made lemonade. Your friends might follow suit.

You can also take the lead on plans, so they don't revolve around drinking. Fact is, your friends might be just as over meeting up for drinks as you are, but everyone's too busy to come up with something better. Host a game night, craft night, a museum trip, bowling, or a pickleball match under the lights. "Anything that uses your hands or your body is fun," while taking the emphasis off drinking, says Gardner.

If your friends bring alcohol? That's fine—and out of your control. What you can control is creating an environment where the main event isn't booze.

4. Confide in trusted friends, and let them know how to support you.

You don't need to announce your drinking habits to everyone, but looping in a few close friends can be a good idea, says Padovano. "Find a believer," she says—someone who is supportive of you. Gardner says you can open the conversation before heading out. Share your goal and what kind of support you're looking for. You can simply say, "Hey, I'm trying to drink less right now," and explain why—if you feel like it.

You might be surprised to learn friends share your sentiment. That solidarity can boost your confidence. If you're worried about pushback while you're out, having an ally is key. "You can even find somebody willing to not drink with you that night," Young says. Whatever you need—subtle backup or a pal to order from the spirit-free section to start—communicate it.

5. Find something else to calm your nerves.

If you feel like alcohol helps you in a social setting, you're not alone. But there are healthier ways to get that same effect, says Gardner. Looking for confidence, a sense of calm, connection? You can get there without the buzz. Instead of pregaming your date with a White Claw, turn on a pump-up playlist to boost your confidence or try a yoga meditation.

Feeling anxious once you arrive? Sneak off to the bathroom for a deep-breathing break. This could also be the perfect moment to text or chat with a friend who knows about your drink-less goals—they can be your personal hype squad.

6. Try a dry challenge.

Going cold turkey might not work for everyone, but taking on a dry challenge with an end date, particularly when your friends are doing it, too, can be a powerful way to reset your relationship with alcohol.

"In some ways, not drinking at all is easier because you take the decision-making out of it," says Padovano. Dry January and Sober October are great times to start, providing the sense of community that many crave. Doing a dry challenge with a friend means you have someone to cheer you on (and vent to, if necessary).

Sober, Single, and Ready to Mingle!

How to get out there without liquid courage.

Dating is *hard*. There's connecting with someone new, picking the location, choosing an outfit, coming up with conversation starters, decoding whether or not to go in for the kiss. If you're used to doing it all with the support of alcohol, the idea of stepping out sober can crank up the anxiety even more. So what happens when you're sober or sober-curious in a world where "Want to grab a drink?" is still the go-to first date move?

First, realize that you're not alone. In fact, 75 percent of Gen Z singles want first dates that aren't centered around alcohol, citing a desire to stay clearheaded and make genuine connections, according to a June 2022 study from the dating app Hinge. Two-thirds of the 3,000 singles surveyed also stated that seeing their date get drunk on the first date is a red flag.

This stat indicates that daters don't want to waste their time, says Scott Schutzman, LMFT, a therapist in New York. "If they go on a date, they want to be sure that who they're meeting is who they really are. They're smart enough to know that alcohol can have an impact on one's behavior and also on one's judgment." He adds that the increase in visibility and awareness for mental illness and addiction might contribute to this mindful dating culture.

Dating without beer (or wine) goggles can be a boon when it comes to judging the quality of your connection. "You are more likely to discover if you truly enjoy spending time with this person without the haze of alcohol, and you are more likely to save time [figuring out if this person is right for you] when you are clear-headed," says Amanda E. White, LPC, licensed therapist and author of *Not Drinking Tonight*.

Regardless of your reasons for abstaining, you may still have questions. Like, how do I keep my nerves in check? How do I tell a Hinge match that wine bars aren't my vibe these days? And what do you even do on a sober date, anyway?

When should I jump into sober dating?

First off, don't rush it. Most folks who are taking a step back from booze can benefit from the notion of dating themselves. Yes, even those in relationships! Whether you take a pottery

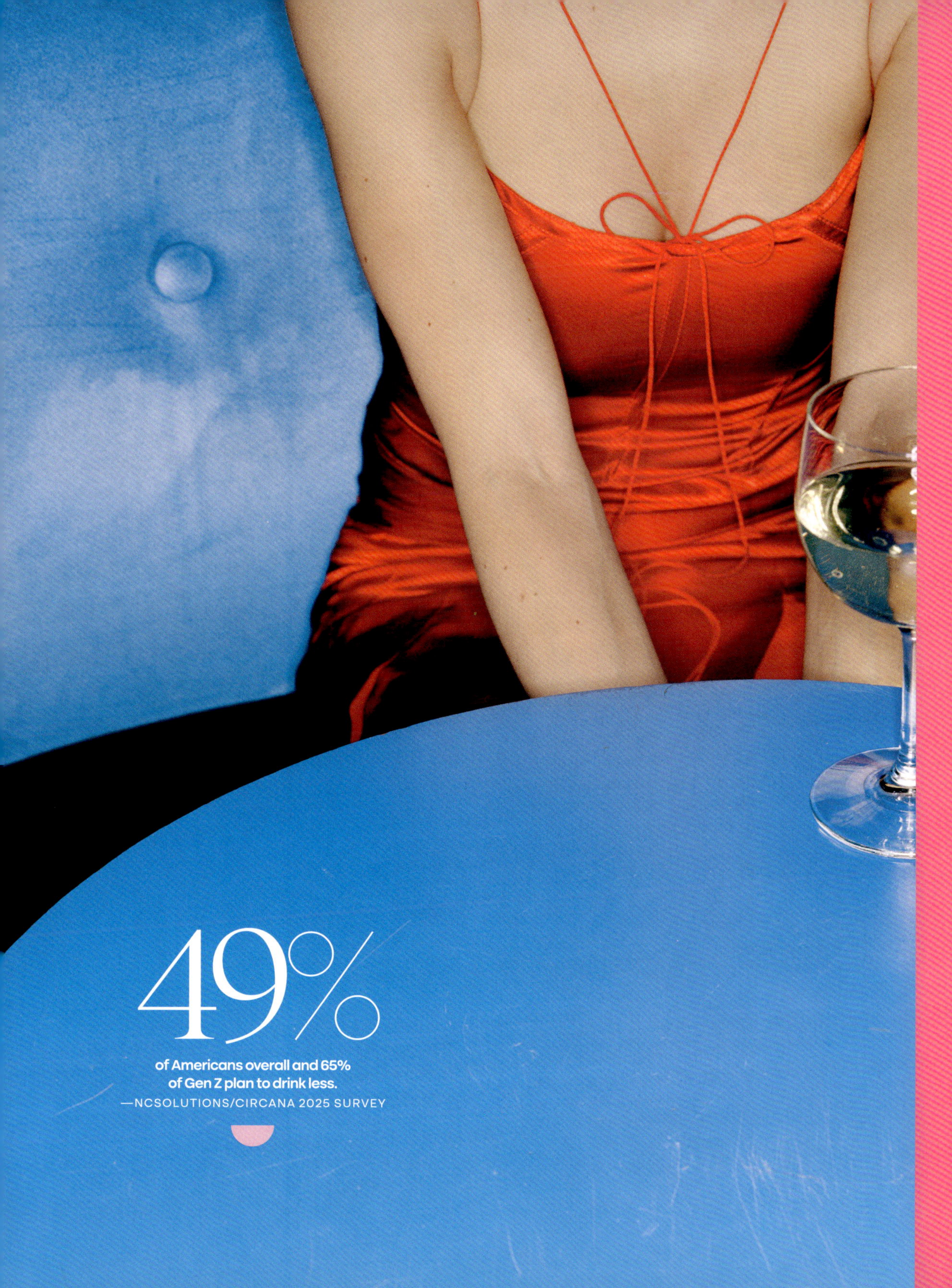
49%
of Americans overall and 65%
of Gen Z plan to drink less.
—NCSOLUTIONS/CIRCANA 2025 SURVEY

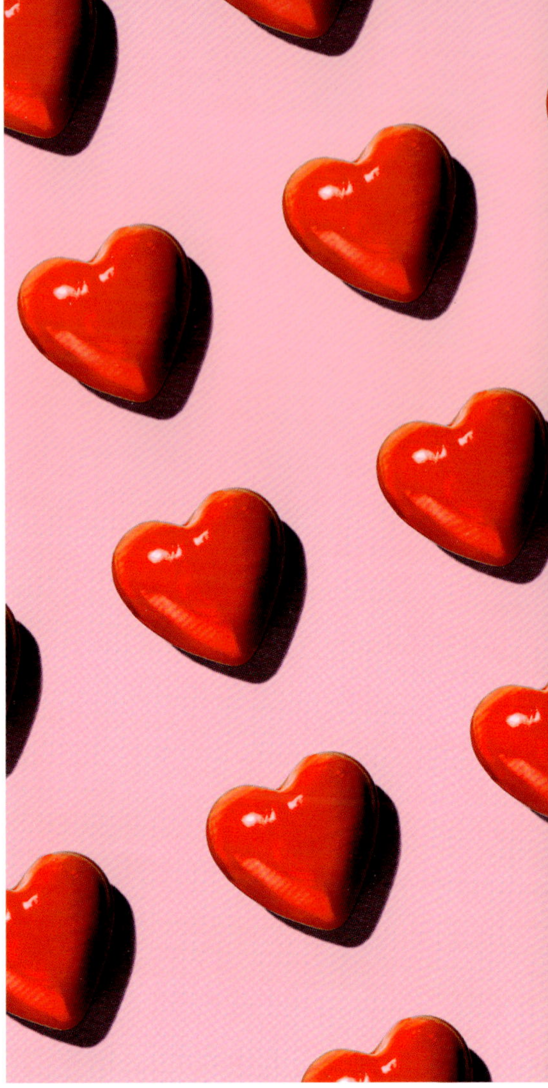

workshop, get into rock climbing, or volunteer for an organization that means something to you, you'll enjoy reconnecting with yourself while also meeting like-minded people. Flexing those creative muscles can also help you feel more confident and connected to the essence of you. Plus, you'll have fun topics to discuss on your dates, when the time comes.

When do I "come out" as sober?

Dating apps make it easier to share your sobriety; Bumble even has a sobriety filter. "Your dating profile is a good place to throw down the info if you want to filter people out," says Bethany Stevens, a sober sex educator getting her PhD in sociology. You may get fewer responses, but they may be better matches.

If you'd rather bring up your sobriety later, try weaving it into your DMs or texts. Try something like, "Hey! Your dog is adorable (or reference something in their photo). Would you two like to go for a walk tomorrow afternoon?" Or, if you're replying to their "Want to grab a drink?" message, try something simple like, "I'd love to! As long as a drink includes mocktails." Then suggest your favorite sober-friendly spot. You can also wait to disclose until you're on the date. Ordering a non-alcoholic drink makes the point without making it a big deal.

When you're ready to share, do so with pride. The decision to abstain from alcohol is a sign of prioritizing your personal, physical, mental, and emotional health, Schutzman adds. And if your date can't respect that? "Then it's simply time to say 'Thank you, take care,' and keep it moving," he says.

What should I do on a sober date?

Spoiler alert: Dating is inherently booze-free! It's up to us if we want to add the wine (or the margaritas or Negronis). One of the best zero-proof antidotes to first-date jitters is doing something playful and active, such as a cooking class, a museum visit, or a game night. It's all about creating an experience, says Keisha Scott, host of *Done with Debauchery,* a sobriety and wellness podcast.

Like any date, a sober date can also end in the bedroom, if you're both comfortable with that. If the thought of hooking up without alcohol makes you nervous, you're not alone. When you are ready to move to that next level, it's important to check in with yourself and your partner about the pace of things.

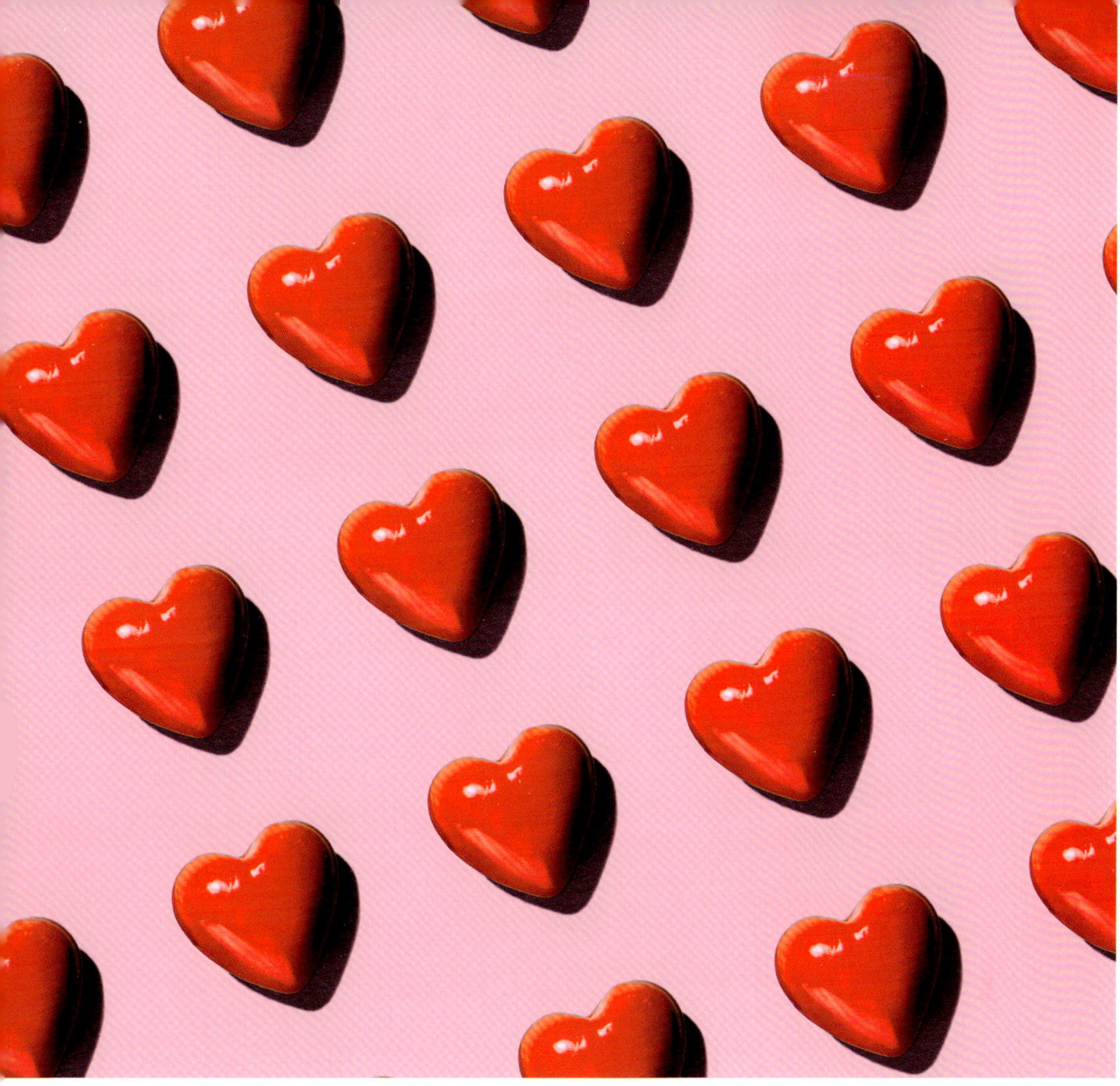

Clear communication with your partner can be an example of building emotional intimacy. "It's important for people to learn the difference between emotional intimacy and physical intimacy," White says. "A lot of people use physical intimacy as a crutch, to avoid their feelings, to avoid having hard conversations, to avoid being honest with themselves or someone else." Saying something like, "This is my first time hooking up without alcohol. I need to take this slow," can set the tone, provide a speed bump, and build your emotional connection, as well.

The Takeaway

Sober dating isn't about knuckling through a million awkward nights: It's about showing up as your truest self. With that kind of clarity, you'll no longer feel the societal pressure to "just grab a drink." Even better—you'll realize you never needed the liquid courage, because you had that confidence inside you all along.

Equip Your Mocktail Cart

Whether you're hosting friends or winding down solo, having ingredients and tools for spirit-free swigs on hand makes it easier to skip the booze. Use this list to stock up, so you'll be ready to deliver a delish, non-alcoholic pour anytime.

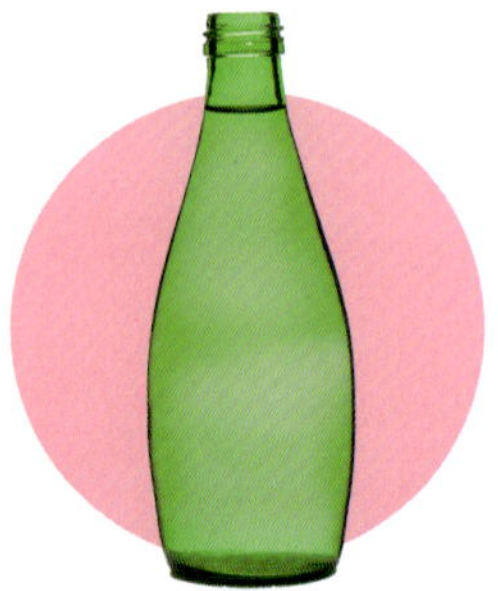

Bubbles + Bases

- ○ **Sparkling Water or Soda Water** It adds lift, fizz, and a sense of occasion. Use it to make spritzes, top off shrubs, and round out sips.
- ○ **Ginger Beer** Pleasingly zingy, it brings depth to mocktails like mules.
- ○ **Flavored Seltzers** Easily add hints of citrus and other fruit to spirit-free bevs by keeping a variety on hand.
- ○ **Club Soda** Crisp and effervescent, it adds bubbles and a clean finish. Its subtle minerality enhances flavors, making it a go-to topper for spritzes and classic highball-style sips.

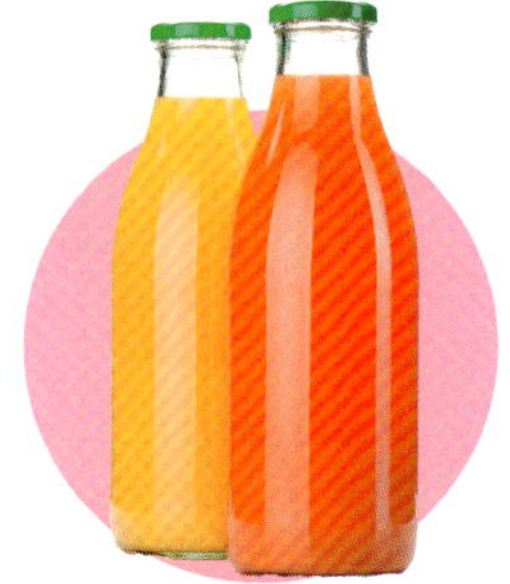

Juices

- ○ **Lime** Its tart, refreshing zing balances out spirit-free drinks. Don't get caught without fresh limes.
- ○ **Lemon** Add brightness and zip to complement everything from berries to botanicals. Keep fresh lemons on hand.
- ○ **Pineapple** Tropical and tangy, this juice brings sweetness, acidity, and a sunny vibe to zero-proof sips.
- ○ **Orange** It can act as a base or a supporting flavor. Level up with fresh oranges, if you'd like.

- ○ **Cranberry** Tart and vibrant, it plays well with citrus, herbs, and bubbles. It's a festive must-have for holiday pours.
- ○ **Tart Cherry** Its deep-red hue and sophisticated tartness pairs well with citrus, vanilla, or spice for a balanced, grown-up sip.
- ○ **Guava Nectar** Thick and tropical, its floral, slightly tangy flavor plays well with lime or coconut, for an island-inspired mocktail.

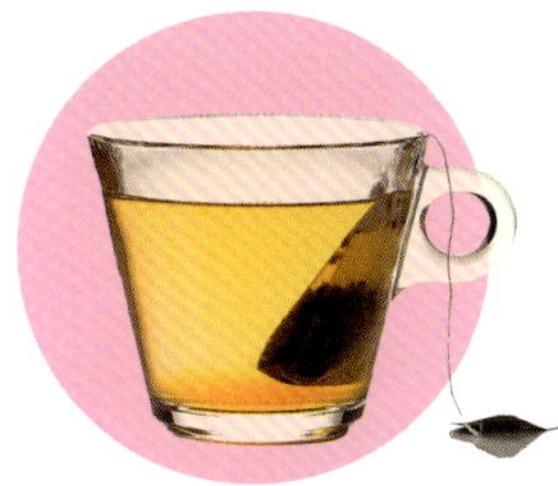

Teas

- ○ **Chamomile** This variety brings floral and herby notes to mocktails, Plus, chamomile is caffeine-free and known for its soothing qualities.
- ○ **Green** This brew (originally Chinese, but also a cornerstone of Japanese culture) lends a light, grassy flavor to tipples, along with antioxidants and a caffeine kick.
- ○ **Black** The tangy tannins in this caffeinated kind of tea adds spine to all sorts of sips.
- ○ **Hibiscus** Tart, red, and naturally caffeine-free, it adds a tang and a cranberry-like hue that enhances a range of drinks.
- ○ **Yerba Mate** This slightly smoky caffeinated herbal tea lends a complex, tea-meets-herb flavor.
- ○ **Hojicha** This mild green tea imparts hints of caramel and hazelnut, and it's low in caffeine, so it won't mess with your sleep.
- ○ **Chai** With notes of cinnamon, cardamom, and clove, it adds cozy depth to mocktails, complementing apple, vanilla, and honey.

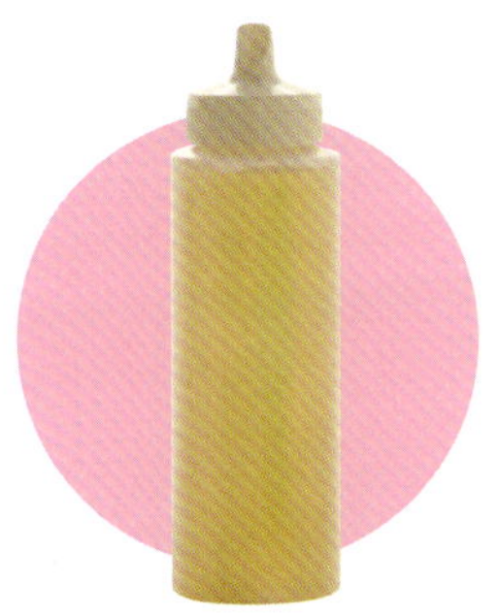

Syrups + Sweeteners

- ○ **Simple Syrup** This liquid sweetener dissolves instantly in cold drinks, like spritzes and sparkling sips, and can be infused with herbs and other flavors. Make your own with the recipe on p. 56.
- ○ **Agave** Made from the agave plant, this natural sweetener has a silky texture similar to that of liquor. It dissolves instantly when stirred into drinks.
- ○ **Grenadine** It adds sweetness and a lovely rosy color to more than just Shirley Temples! Make your own with the recipe on p. 75.
- ○ **Orgeat Syrup** Made from almonds and orange flower water (sometimes along with cinnamon, cloves, and vanilla), it imparts a creamy, nutty taste.
- ○ **Maple Syrup** Rich and velvety, pure maple syrup brings warmth and depth while blending easily into cold drinks.
- ○ **Honey** Add natural sweetness with a touch of complexity to citrus, tea-based, and herbal swills. It blends best when warmed or mixed into a syrup first.
- ○ **Cream of Coconut** Indulgently tropical, cream of coconut adds sweetness, richness, and body. It blends best with citrus or pineapple juices, evoking vacation-ready vibes.
- ○ **Calamansi Syrup** This sweet-and-sour syrup is made from the calamansi, a small Asian citrus fruit. It delivers a tropical zip and a punch that sits between lime and mandarin.
- ○ **Passionfruit Syrup** Lush, tart, and exotic, it brings tropical intensity to spritzes, sours, and other fruit-forward mocktails.
- ○ **Lemongrass Syrup** Its bright, slightly floral notes pair beautifully with ginger, coconut, or lime, bringing freshness to any drink.

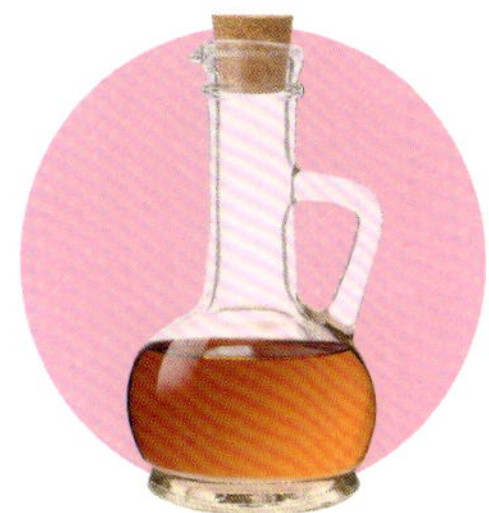

Vinegars

- ○ **Apple Cider Vinegar** Tart and fruity, this adds a bite to shrubs. Its sweetness and fermented tang straddle the line between sweet and sour for a crisp-tasting sip.
- ○ **Rice Vinegar** Delicate, mellow, and subtly sweet, it brings gentle acidity to a shrub without overpowering. It smooths out sharper fruits and herbs, creating a clean, balanced base that lets other flavors shine.
- ○ **Balsamic Vinegar** Rich and tangy with a touch of sweetness, just a drizzle can bring depth to mules or fruit-based drinks.

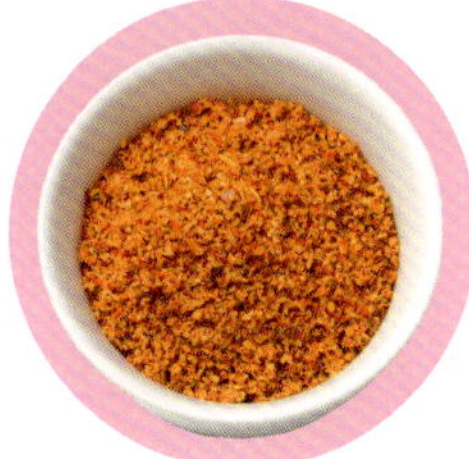

Rimmers + Garnishes

- ○ **Tajín** This chile-lime salt blend gives spicy mocktails an extra kick—and looks great on a rimmed glass.

○ **Coarse Kosher Salt** It clings well to a lime-rimmed glass and lends a satisfying crunch.

○ **Luxardo Cherries** Keep a jar of these marasca cherries, candied using a process without artificial colors and flavors, on hand. They're the jewel on top of any drink.

○ **Pomegranate Seeds** They add a burst of sweetness, pleasing crunch, and a festive flourish to tipples.

○ **Candied Ginger** It adds spicy sweetness to drinks, and a pleasing chewiness, too.

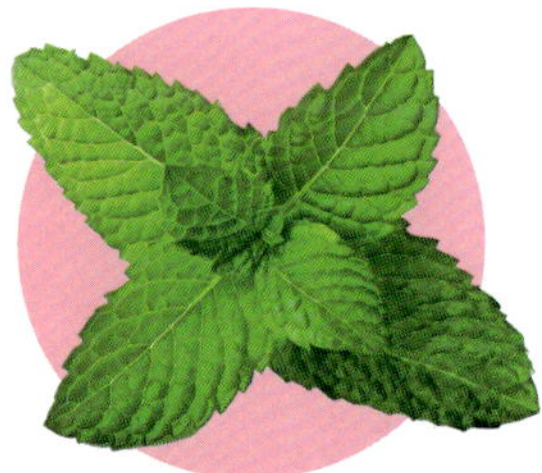

Flavor Enhancers + Bitters

○ **Mint** It gives drinks the essence of freshness, whether muddled or used as a garnish.

○ **Ginger** Use it muddled, juiced, or as a spicy infusion.

○ **Rosemary** Piney and aromatic, it gives zero-proof sips a savory edge.

○ **Non-Alcoholic Bitters** Just a few drops add intrigue with notes of orange peel and spice.

○ **Thyme** Earthy thyme lends subtle herbal complexity to libations. Use a sprig to infuse syrups or muddle it to release its woodsy aroma.

○ **Basil** It adds garden-fresh flavor. Muddle it to release its peppery-sweet notes, or use a sprig as a garnish to complement fruit, citrus, and herbal ingredients.

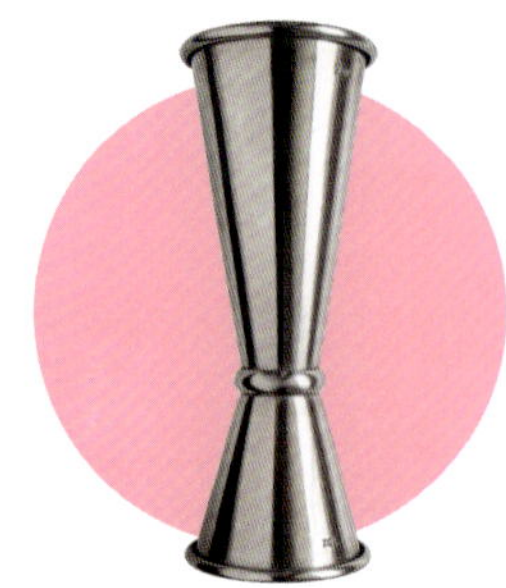

Tools

○ **Shaker** For swigs that need to be chilled and mixed thoroughly, you'll be reaching for this tool on the reg.

○ **Jigger** This dual-sized tool is your go-to for pouring measurements. Get one with 1- and 2-ounce sides to use with the recipes in this book.

○ **Muddler** Use it to extract the oils and flavors from herbs and fruits.

○ **Strainer** Keep seeds, pulp, and herbs out of your finished drink.

○ **Bar Spoon** Use it to stir bubbly drinks without flattening the fizz.

○ **Citrus Press** This handheld tool extracts more juice with less mess.

○ **Fine-Mesh Sieve** This tool is ideal for double-straining shaken drinks.

○ **Cocktail Picks** These petite skewers are designed for propping up a garnish.

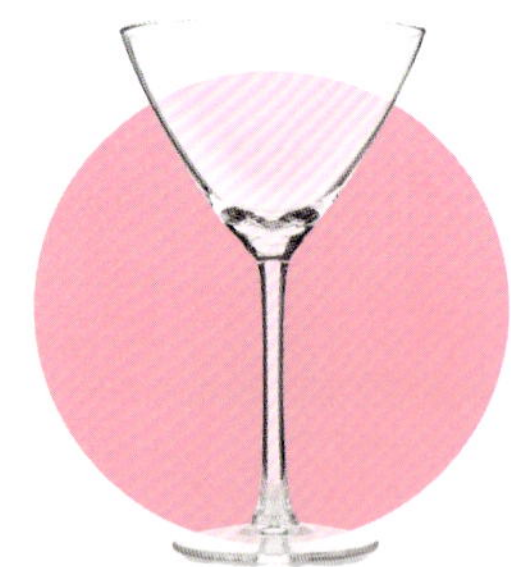

Go-To Glassware

○ **Rocks** Short and sturdy, this is your go-to vessel for drinks served over ice.

○ **Stemless Wine** These also work well for spritzes and shrubs.

○ **Coupe** Elegant and shallow with a wide bowl, it's ideal for shaken sips and anything that feels a little special.

○ **Martini** With its iconic V shape, it suits cocktails that are crisp, clean, and served straight up.

○ **Highball** Tall and straight-sided, it's perfect for fizzy drinks.

○ **Collins** Slightly taller than a highball, this glass works well for long, ice-filled swigs that build in layers, like spritzes and shrubs.

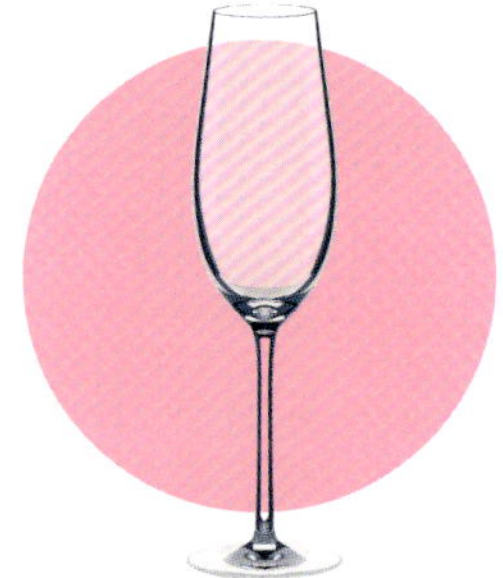

Nice-To-Have Glassware

○ **Champagne Flute** Tall and slender, this glass preserves bubbles beautifully.

○ **Copper Mug** The classic cup for mules, it keeps drinks icy-cold.

○ **Mason Jar** It's a vintage vessel for casual, fruity sips.

○ **Nick and Nora** This is a smaller cousin to the coupe, built for a compact pour.

○ **Tulip** Its bulbous body (like the flower) traps aromas, making it ideal for sips that benefit from a strong nose, like complex mocktails. The stem keeps your hand from warming the drink.

○ **Margarita** Its shape showcases colorful margs, and an extra-wide rim lets you savor more salty slugs.

○ **Sling** Tall and narrow, this elegant glass puts long, layered, bubbly sips on display.

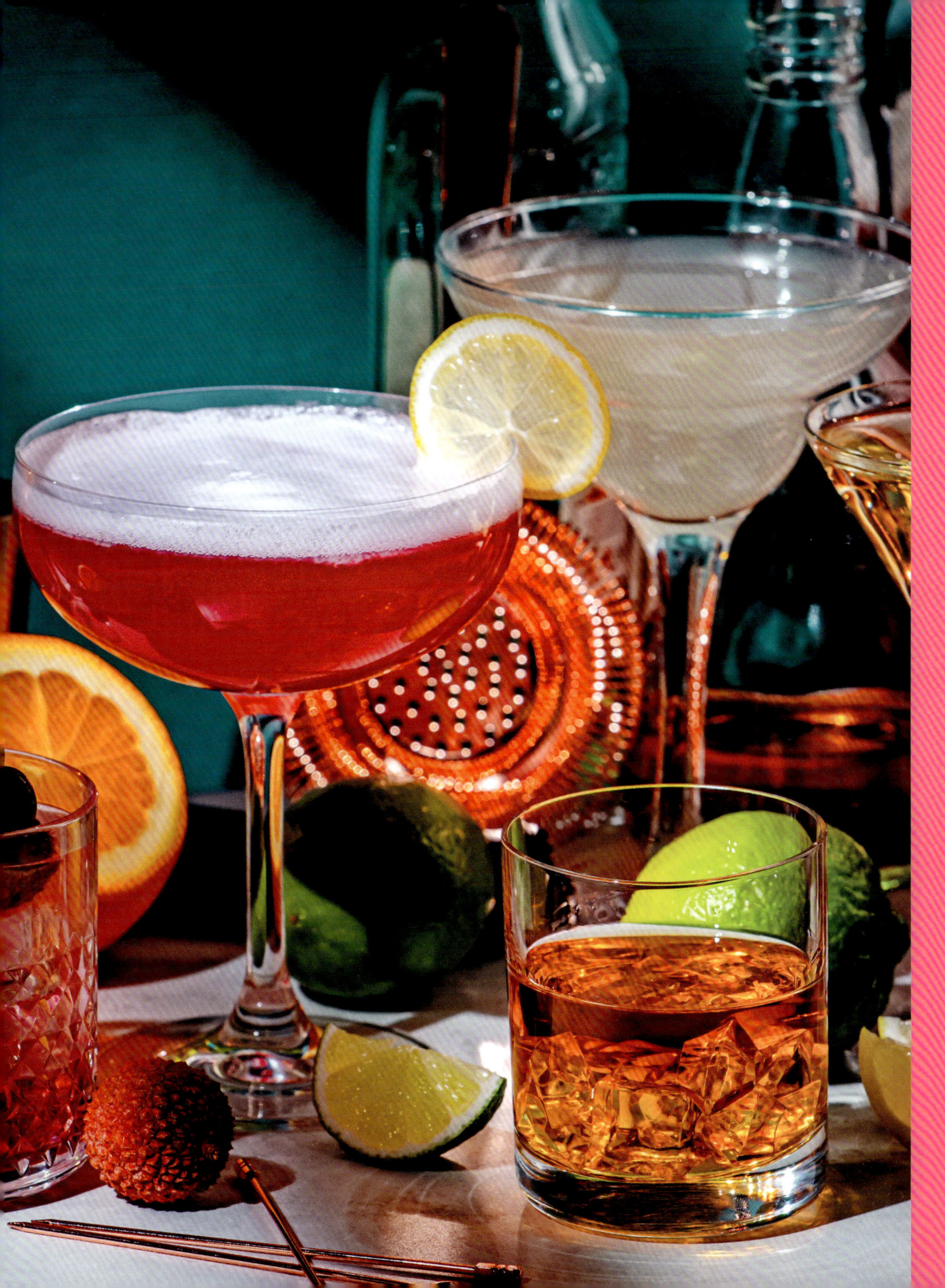

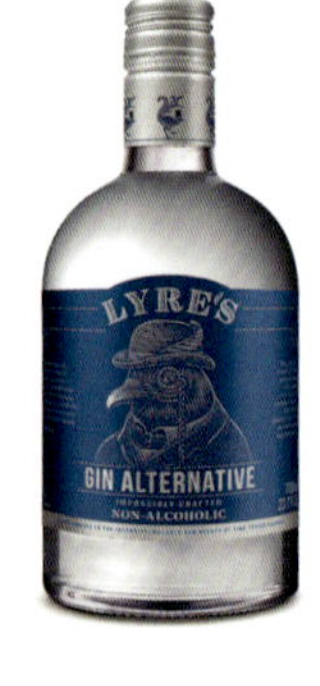

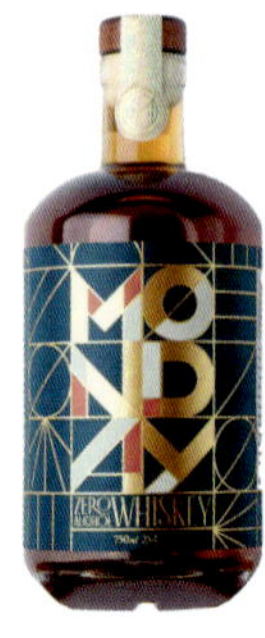

Stock Up!

You don't need an array of bottles to turn out spirit-free sips. Start with staples; add to your stash over time.

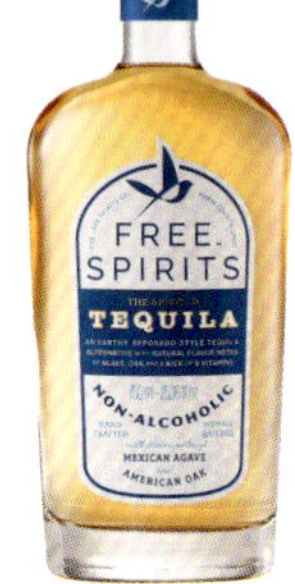

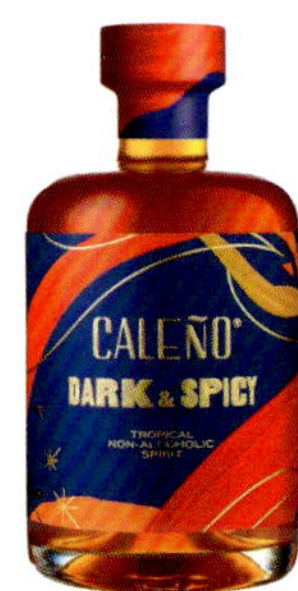

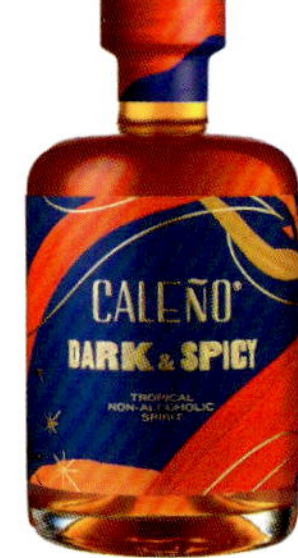

STAPLES

You'll definitely want these workhorses on hand. The labels we've called out rank well with our favorite mixologists.

Spirit-Free Gin

Lyre's Gin Alternative

Botanical and crisp, this pour brings floral and herbal structure to spritzes. In the style of a good London dry gin, this alternative leads with piney juniper notes, supported by orange blossom and citrus.

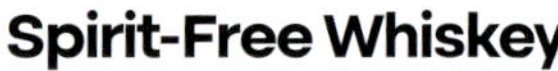

Spirit-Free Whiskey

Monday Zero Alcohol Whiskey

Warm and woody, this spirit alternative serves as the backbone of old-fashioneds, Manhattans, and whiskey sours. This version has the aroma of butterscotch, raisin, and toasted brown sugar, and the taste of coffee, caramel, and molasses, with a little heat, too.

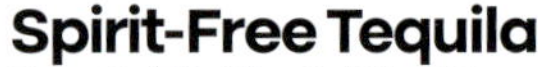

Spirit-Free Tequila

Free Spirits The Spirit of Tequila

Herbaceous, peppery, and dry, non-alc tequila is the choice for margaritas, palomas, citrus coolers, and spicy sips. This particular label is crafted from Mexican blue agave, offering a complex flavor rivaling traditional reposado.

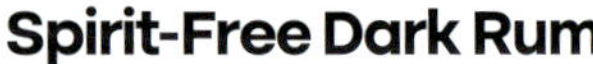

Spirit-Free Dark Rum

Caleño Dark & Spicy Tropical Rum Alternative

This amber-hued spirit alternative evokes the sun-drenched flavors of Colombia (the founder's family homeland), with its notes of molasses and sultry baking spices.

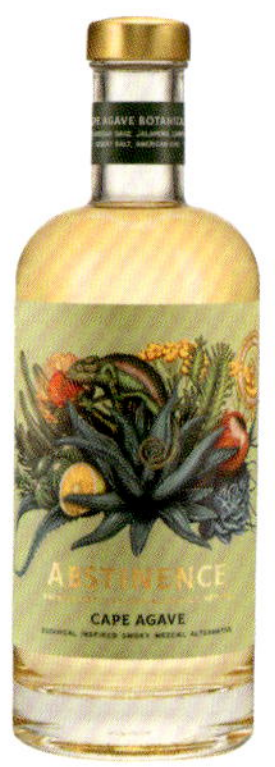

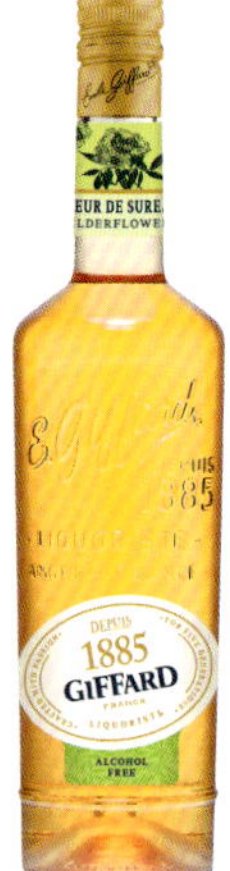

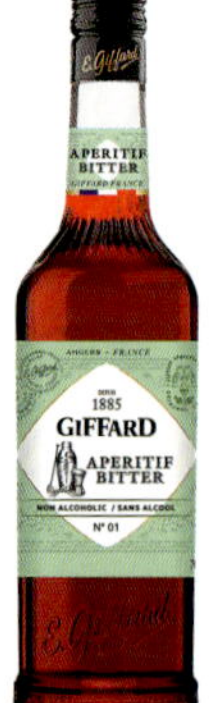

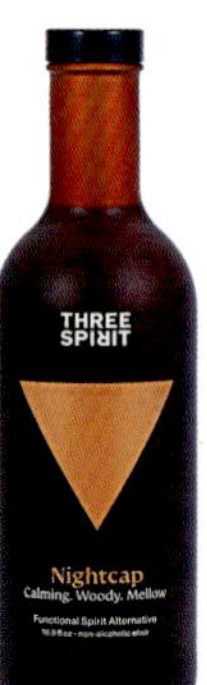

NICE-TO-HAVES

Looking to level up? Round out your offerings with these sips.

Spirit-Free Mezcal

Abstinence Cape Agave

Smoky, earthy, and complex, mezcal is a go-to for citrusy margs, palomas, or sophisticated sips, such as the Hopeless Pyromantic (p. 132). Tequila is one type of mezcal, and it must be made with at least 51% blue Weber agave; mezcal can be crafted from other varieties of agave. This particular non-alc mezcal is made with sage, arabica bean, mesquite, jalapeño, and agave.

Spirit-Free Elderflower Liqueur

Giffard Elderflower

Fragrant and floral, this spirit imparts a soft sweetness and perfume of summer blooms to light mocktails, like the Char Bear (p. 86) and Peach Blossom (p. 140). This zero-proof version, made from elderflower blossoms macerated in white wine vinegar, tastes of lychee, rose, and wormwood.

Spirit-Free Energizing Botanical

Three Spirit Livener

This spiced elixir combines the herbs guayusa, schisandra, and ginseng for a natural lift. Its berry flavor and touch of heat make it an intriguing base for spritzes, including the Bayberry Spritz (p. 128), or citrus-based mocktails.

Spirit-Free Herbal Soother

Three Spirit Nightcap

A woodsy blend of valerian root, hops, and lemon balm. With notes of maple, vanilla, and spice, it's delish in Kava & Chill (p. 127). Or sip it neat or with a splash of soda over ice to unwind.

Spirit-Free Italian Aperitif

Giffard Aperitif Bitter

This non-alcoholic red syrup can stand in for classic Italian bitter liqueurs like Campari or Aperol. Add a splash to club soda for a simple, refreshing sipper. With notes of orange peel and herbs, it brings a pleasantly bitter, citrus-forward spine to spritzes. Try it in a Freebird (p. 93) or add a splash to soda water for ruby-hued refreshment.

Wine Time!

Non-alcoholic vinos can be hit-or-miss, but these labels make the grade with the pros.

- **NA Sparkling White**

Moderato La Cuvée Révolutionnaire Colombard

Made with Colombard grapes from Gascony, a region in Southwest France near the Pyrenees, this pour is aromatic with pears and peaches, acidic, and celebration-worthy. It's lovely on its own or in a spritz, like the Spring in Kyoto (p. 77).

- **NA Sparkling Rose**

French Bloom Le Rosé Alcohol-Free Sparkling Wine

If it didn't say so on the bottle, you may not even know the alcohol has been removed from this refreshing sparkling French rosé. It's got everything you'd expect in its boozy counterpart: minerality, tasty fruit notes, and good acidity.

- **NA White**

Proxie Blanc Slate

This wine alternative sings with citrus and stone fruit. It features sauvignon grapes along with kiwi, apricot, and grapefruit concentrate, and white peony tea, for a multi-dimensional sip that's worthy of special occasions but also delicious with everyday dinners.

- **NA Red**

Thomson Scott Noughty Rouge Non Alcoholic

This balanced, semi-dry sip gets high marks from picky palates and sober bartenders, who prize its nose, flavor, and similar-to-the-real-thing mouth feel. Enjoy it with a big meal, or on the sofa after dinner.

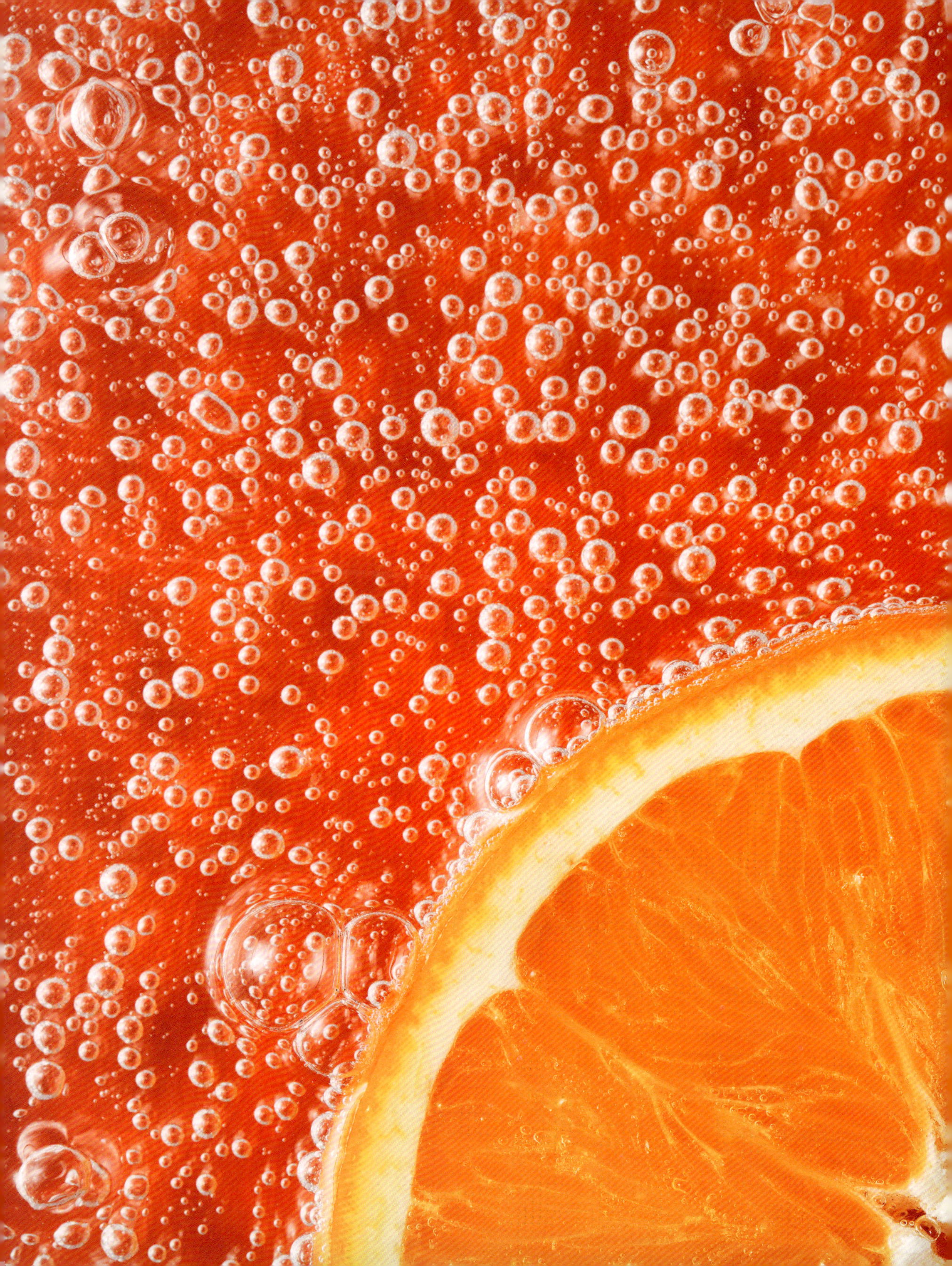

CHAPTER TWO

Cheers to Everyday Sparkle!

» With this slew of 50 simple, satisfying, spirit-free drink recipes from master mixologists, you can savor a delightful tipple (or two) while staying true to your wellness goals.

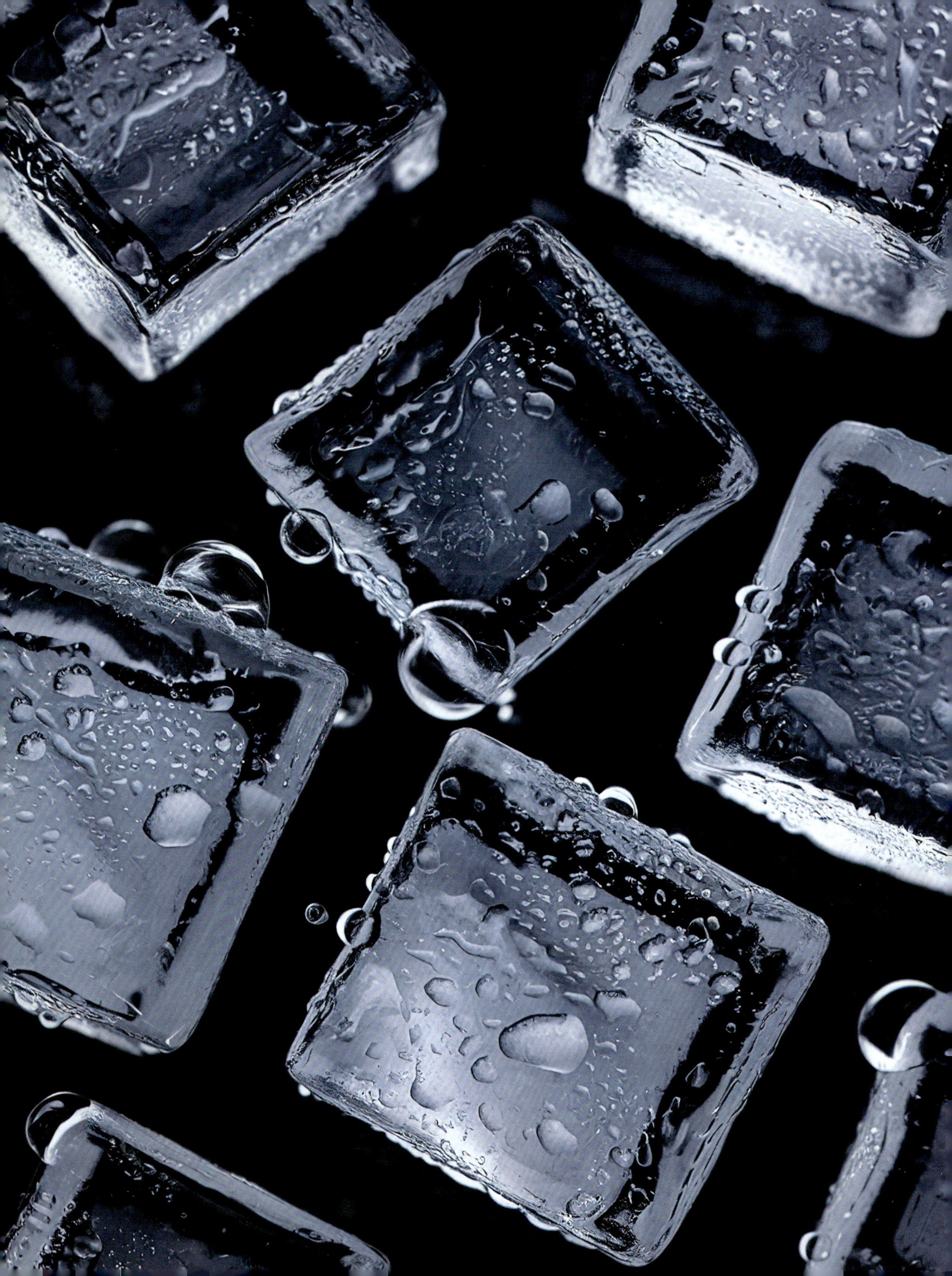

THE JOYS OF GOING SOBERISH

At *Women's Health*, we've watched as the culture around alcohol and drinking has shifted drastically in the past few years—particularly within the health and wellness sphere. We know that Gen Z is drinking less than ever before, but they're not the only ones: Interest in mocktails, zero-proof spirits, and an alcohol-free lifestyle has surged among our audience, including women of all ages.

However, our readers are also looking for ways to still enjoy the social and flavor perks of cocktail culture...sans the cocktail. That's where this book comes in: We're sharing our absolute favorite recipes—meticulously developed and tested by our test kitchen editors—as well as some of the most creative and delicious mocktails you'll find from bartenders around the country, from New York City to Los Angeles. Some of these mixologists work at alcohol-free establishments like Lil Deb's Oasis in Hudson, New York, and female-owned bars like the Velveteen Rabbit in Las Vegas.

The best part is that the spirit-free recipes shared in the pages ahead are easy enough to mix up in your own home, yet exciting to sip, featuring innovative ingredients and new techniques that offer complex flavor profiles. (You'll feel like you're at the trendiest new bar—right at your kitchen counter, promise.)

In addition to the drinks themselves, you'll also find inspiring stories from people who have reduced or eliminated alcohol from their lives—and how doing so has boosted their health, happiness, and sense of connection. We've also highlighted recipes that are lower in added sugar (defined as 10 grams or fewer of sugar per serving) and included nutritional information throughout, so you can make mindful choices while enjoying every flavorful pour.

Because you can have your healthy fun *and* drink it, too.

Abigail Cuffey,
Executive Editor, *Women's Health*

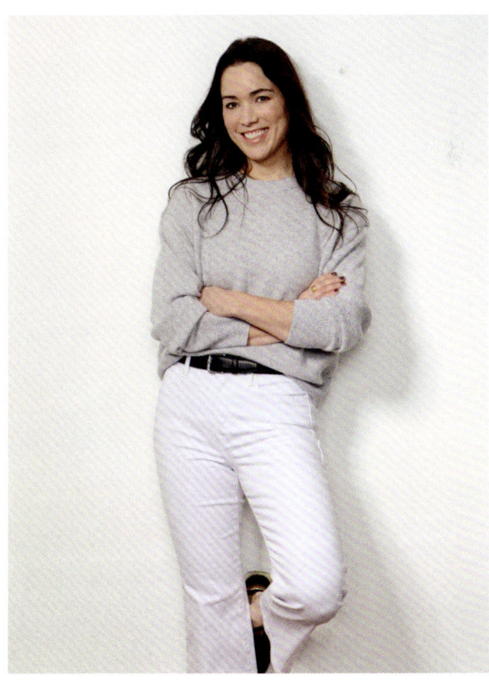

Spritzers and Shrubs

Fizz and fruit define these drinks.

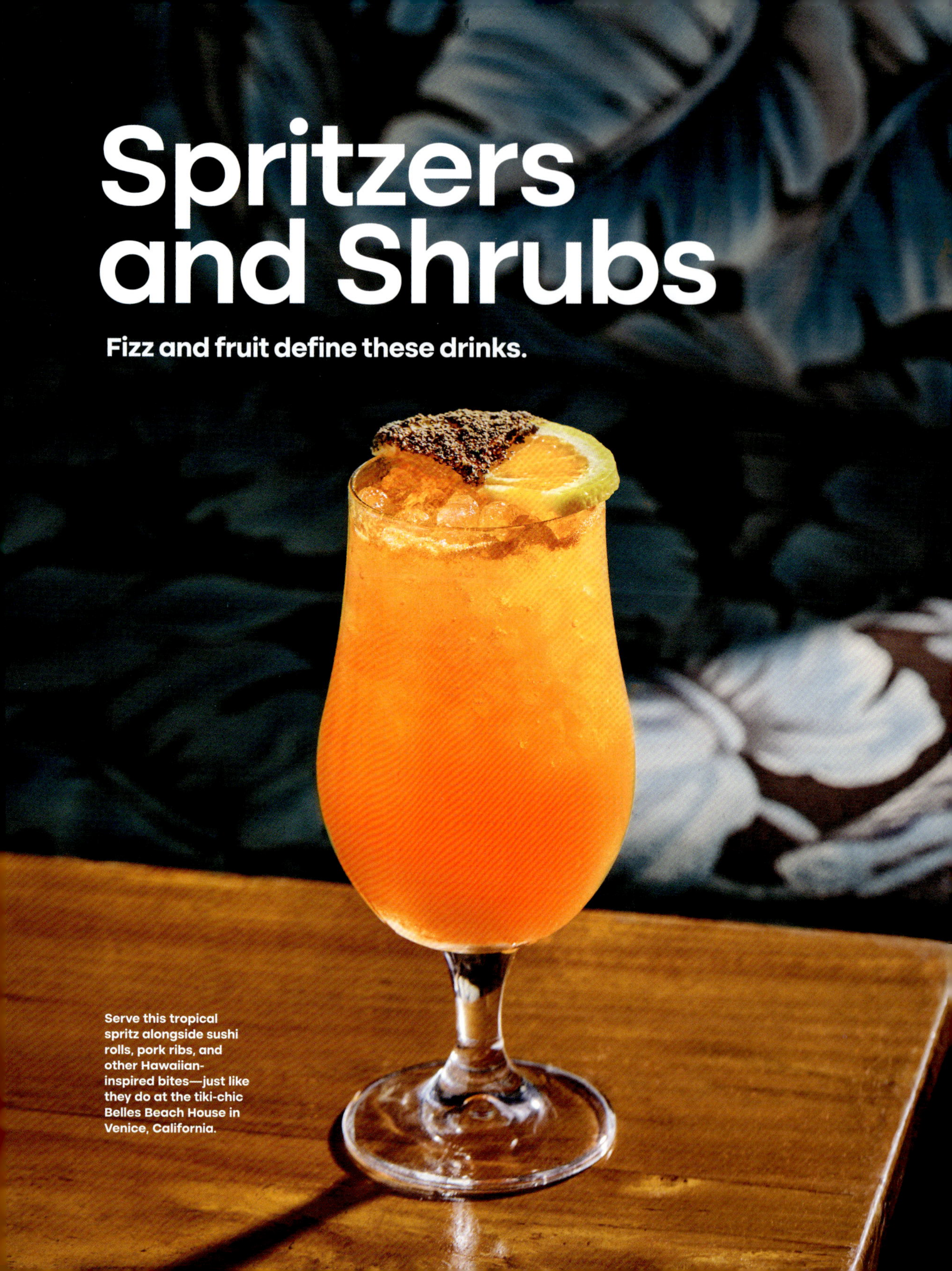

Serve this tropical spritz alongside sushi rolls, pork ribs, and other Hawaiian-inspired bites—just like they do at the tiki-chic Belles Beach House in Venice, California.

Staycation Spritz

- **4** oz sparkling water
- **3/4** oz carrot juice
- **3/4** oz orange juice
- **3/4** oz lemon juice
- **1/4** oz turmeric juice
- **3/4** oz Agave Syrup (recipe below)
- Ice, for shaking and serving
- Orange slice dipped in black pepper, for serving

1. Pour 4 oz sparkling water into 12- to 16-oz glass, such as a tulip glass.

2. In shaker, combine juices and Agave Syrup. Add a few ice cubes and shake 5 to 10 seconds. Strain over the sparkling water, then add ice. Garnish with an orange slice dipped in black pepper.

Serves 1. Per serving: About 73 cal, 0 g fat, (0 g sat fat), 0 mg chol, 37 mg sodium, 18.5 g carb, 0 g fiber, 13 g sugar, (9.5 g added sugar), 0 g pro

INGREDIENT EXPLAINER

Turmeric juice, an orange-colored extract from the turmeric root, contains curcumin, an antioxidant that may ease inflammation and support the immune system. You can buy turmeric juice in the form of a "wellness shot" at Trader Joe's, Whole Foods, and specialty markets.

Agave Syrup

MIX equal parts agave and water (e.g., 1/2 cup each). **STIR** in bowl or shake in glass until fully combined. If it's too thick or separating, gently warm it in saucepan over low heat (do not boil), stirring until fully blended. If heated, let cool before using or storing. **STORE** in clean bottle or jar with a lid in the fridge for up to 3 weeks.

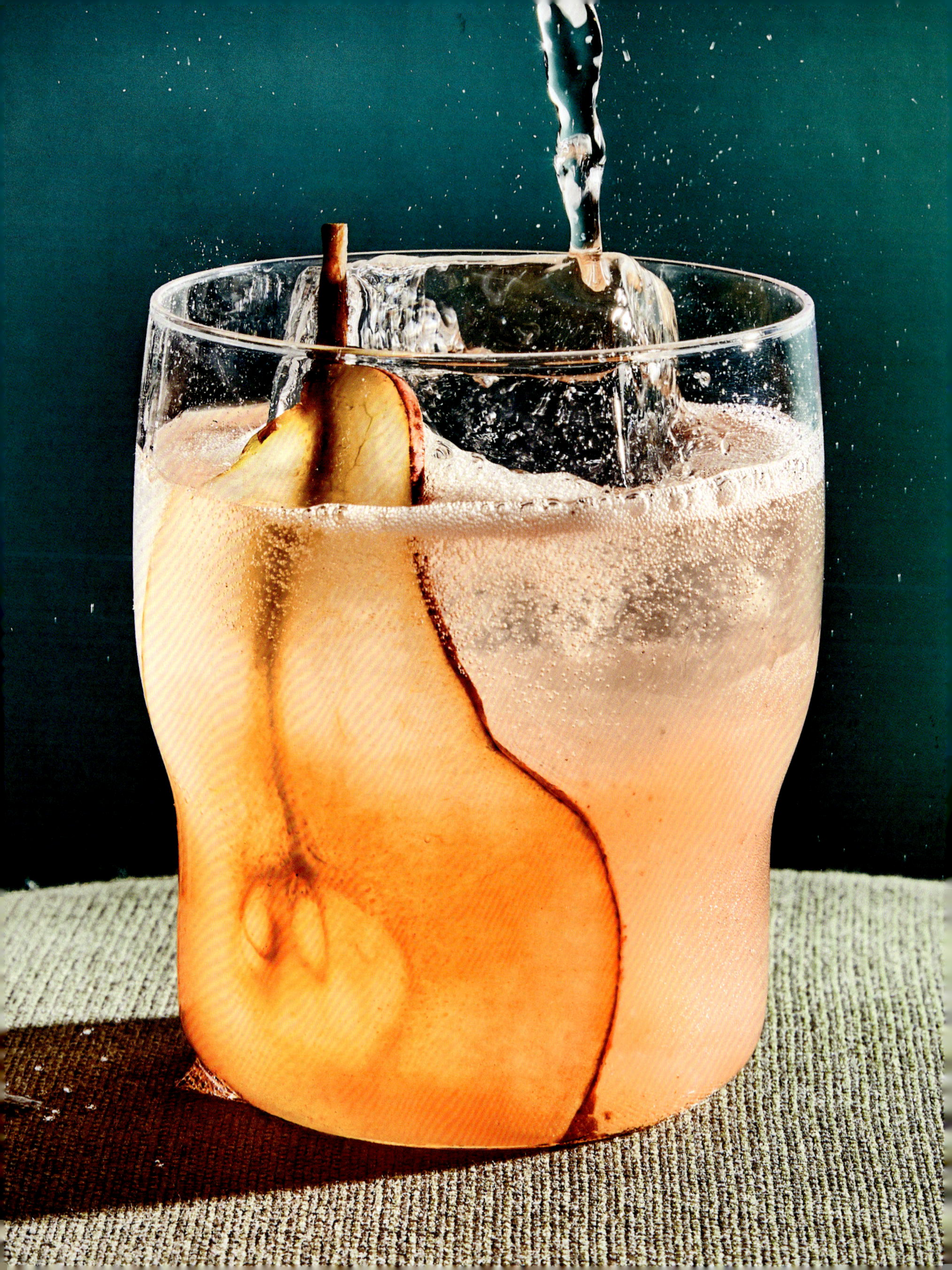

Red Pear Shrub Spritzer

- **1/3** cup sugar
- **1** vanilla bean, split lengthwise
- **5** cardamom pods
- **1** lb (about 2) ripe red pears, roughly chopped, plus pear slices for serving
- **6** Tbsp apple cider vinegar
- Ice, for serving
- Club soda, chilled, for topping off

1 In saucepan, bring ½ cup water, sugar, vanilla, and cardamom to a boil.

2 Add chopped pears, reduce heat, and simmer for 10 minutes, then let stand for 30 minutes. Strain into a jar and stir in vinegar. Refrigerate until cold.

3 If desired, line 2 glasses with pear slices. Add ice. Divide shrub between glasses (½ cup in each) and top with club soda.

Serves 2. Per serving: About 169 cal, 0 g fat (0 g sat), 0 mg chol, 16 mg sodium, 41 g carb, 1 g fiber, 38.5 g sugar (33 g added sugar), 0 g pro

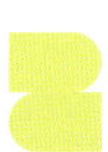

PRO TIP Swap the pears for whatever fruit is in season; berries, apples, and citrus are fair game. This sip is built on a shrub—a tangy mix of fruit, sugar, and vinegar—which not only adds zing but may support digestion and gut health.

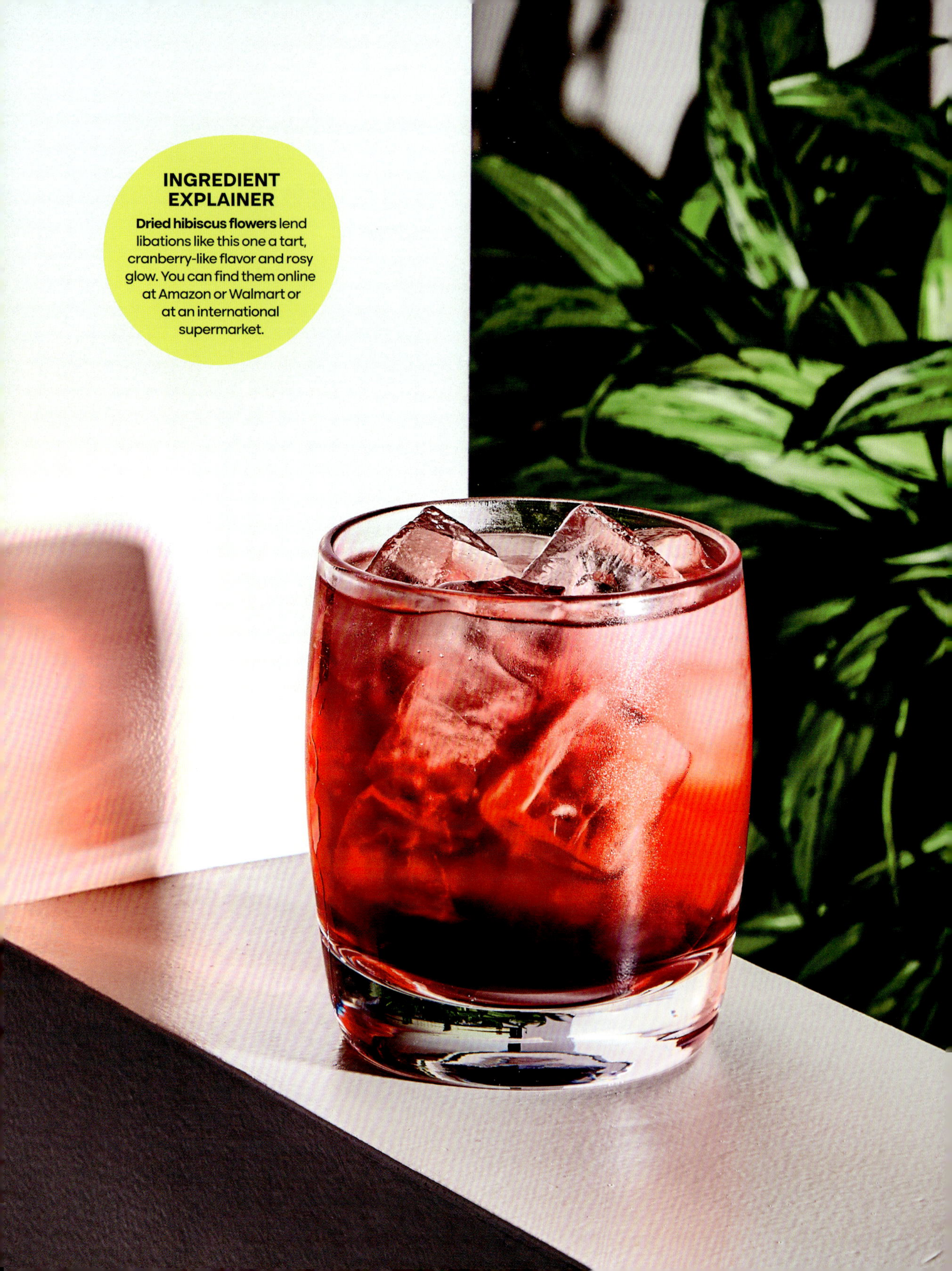
INGREDIENT EXPLAINER
Dried hibiscus flowers lend libations like this one a tart, cranberry-like flavor and rosy glow. You can find them online at Amazon or Walmart or at an international supermarket.

LOW-SUGAR SIPPER!

Ginger Hibiscus Spritzer

- **1** 2-inch piece fresh ginger, sliced
- **6** Tbsp loose dried hibiscus flowers
- **3** Tbsp agave
- Ice, for serving
- Club soda, chilled, for topping off

1 In saucepan, bring 1 cup water, ginger, hibiscus flowers, and agave to a boil. Reduce heat and simmer for 5 minutes. Remove from heat and let stand for 10 minutes. Strain the mixture into a pitcher.

2 Stir in 2 cups cold water. For each serving, pour ¼ cup syrup into an ice-filled glass and top with club soda.

Serves 8. Per serving: About 23 cal, 0 g fat (0 g sat), 0 mg chol, 4 mg sodium, 6 g carb, 0 g fiber, 6 g sugar (6 g added sugar), 0 g pro

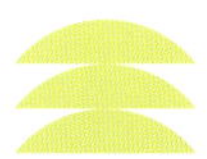

LIFE AFTER ALCOHOL: "Living in line with my values"

Ray decided to stop drinking in 2023 after she finished graduate school. Alcohol was holding her back, she noticed, even in small and infrequent quantities. The exhaustion and lack of energy weren't worth it to her, nor was the ideological disconnect. "I felt like my beliefs and actions were out of sync, as a personal trainer and health advocate," she says. "I've always maintained that you can have a fun and fulfilling life without alcohol, and I realized that if I truly believed that, I should be able to live it. Two years in, I have no regrets!"

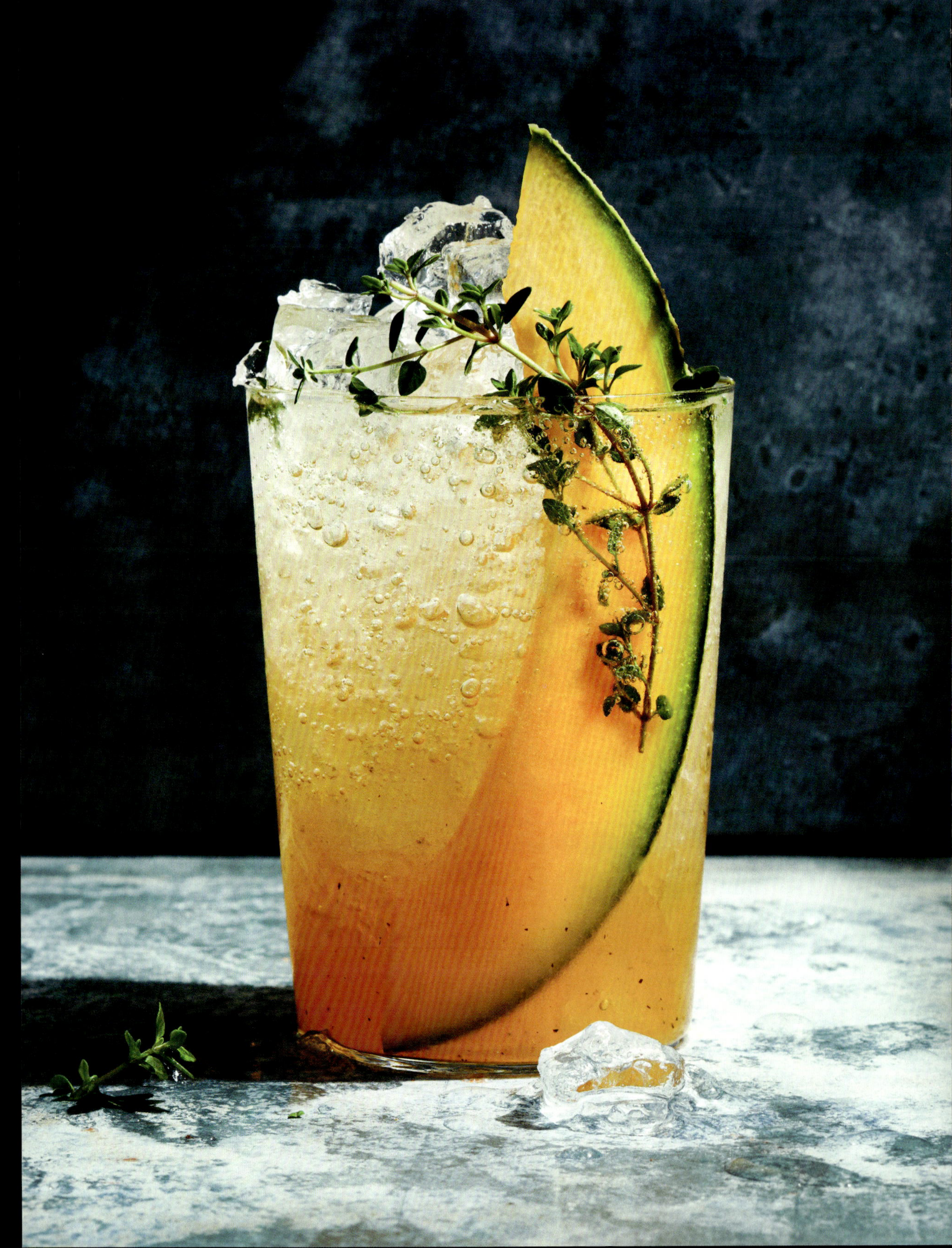

Cantaloupe Thyme Spritzer

- **3** Tbsp Cantaloupe Thyme Shrub (recipe below)
- **½** cup sparkling water, chilled
- Ice, for serving
- Thin cantaloupe wedge and/or thyme sprig, for serving, if desired

Fill tall glass with ice and add Cantaloupe Thyme Shrub and sparkling water. Garnish with cantaloupe wedge and thyme sprig, if desired.

Serves 1. Per serving: About 86 cal, 0 g fat, (0 g sat fat), 0 mg chol, 30.5 mg sodium, 21 g carb, 0 g fiber, 21 g sugar, (19 g added sugar), 0 g pro

PREP AHEAD The Cantaloupe Thyme Shrub is the aromatic backbone of this mocktail. It's also a tasty way to rescue an overripe melon. Store the shrub in jar in the fridge, and it'll keep for a month (or more). Just pour over ice, add bubbles, and enjoy!

Cantaloupe Thyme Shrub

CUT 1 medium cantaloupe (about 2½ lbs), rind and seeds discarded, into 1½-inch pieces (about 3 cups). **COMBINE** cantaloupe, 1½ cups sugar, and 8 thyme sprigs in an airtight container, then smash thyme slightly. **REFRIGERATE,** mixing and smashing twice a day for 2 to 3 days, until flavors are infused. **REMOVE** thyme sprigs. **BLEND** mixture with 1 cup rice vinegar until smooth. Strain through a fine-mesh sieve into a pitcher. **MAKES 3 CUPS** (enough to make 16 cocktails)

FLAVOR PROFILE Made with cooling cucumbers and tart lime juice, this sipper has a botanical intrigue reminiscent of gin, thanks to chilled chamomile tea.

Garden Party Mocktail

- **8** chamomile tea bags
- **½** cup sugar
- **1** English cucumber
- **2** strips lime zest plus 2 lime wheels, for serving
- **½** cup fresh lime juice
- Ice, for shaking and serving
- **12** oz club soda, chilled
- **2** thyme sprigs, for serving

1. In small saucepan, bring 1 cup water to a boil. Remove from heat. Add tea bags and sugar, and stir until sugar dissolves. Let steep for 10 minutes. Strain, squeezing tea bags, into liquid measuring cup; discard tea bags. Let tea cool to room temperature, about 15 minutes.

2. Meanwhile, cut 4 round slices from cucumber and set aside. Using vegetable peeler, thinly shave 4 lengthwise slices from remaining cucumber (you will have cucumber left over). Arrange cucumber ribbons inside 2 tall glasses (at least 16 oz each). Transfer glasses to the freezer.

3. In large shaker, muddle lime zest and reserved round cucumber slices with 2 oz cooled chamomile tea. Add lime juice and remaining chamomile tea; fill shaker with ice and shake until shaker is frosty.

4. Add ice to prepared glasses. Strain mocktail into prepared glasses and gently stir in club soda. Garnish with lime wheels and thyme sprigs.

Serves 2. Per serving: About 68 cal, 0 g fat, (0 g sat fat), 0 mg chol, 41 mg sodium, 18.5 g carb, 0 g fiber, 14 g sugar, (13 g added sugar), 0 g pro

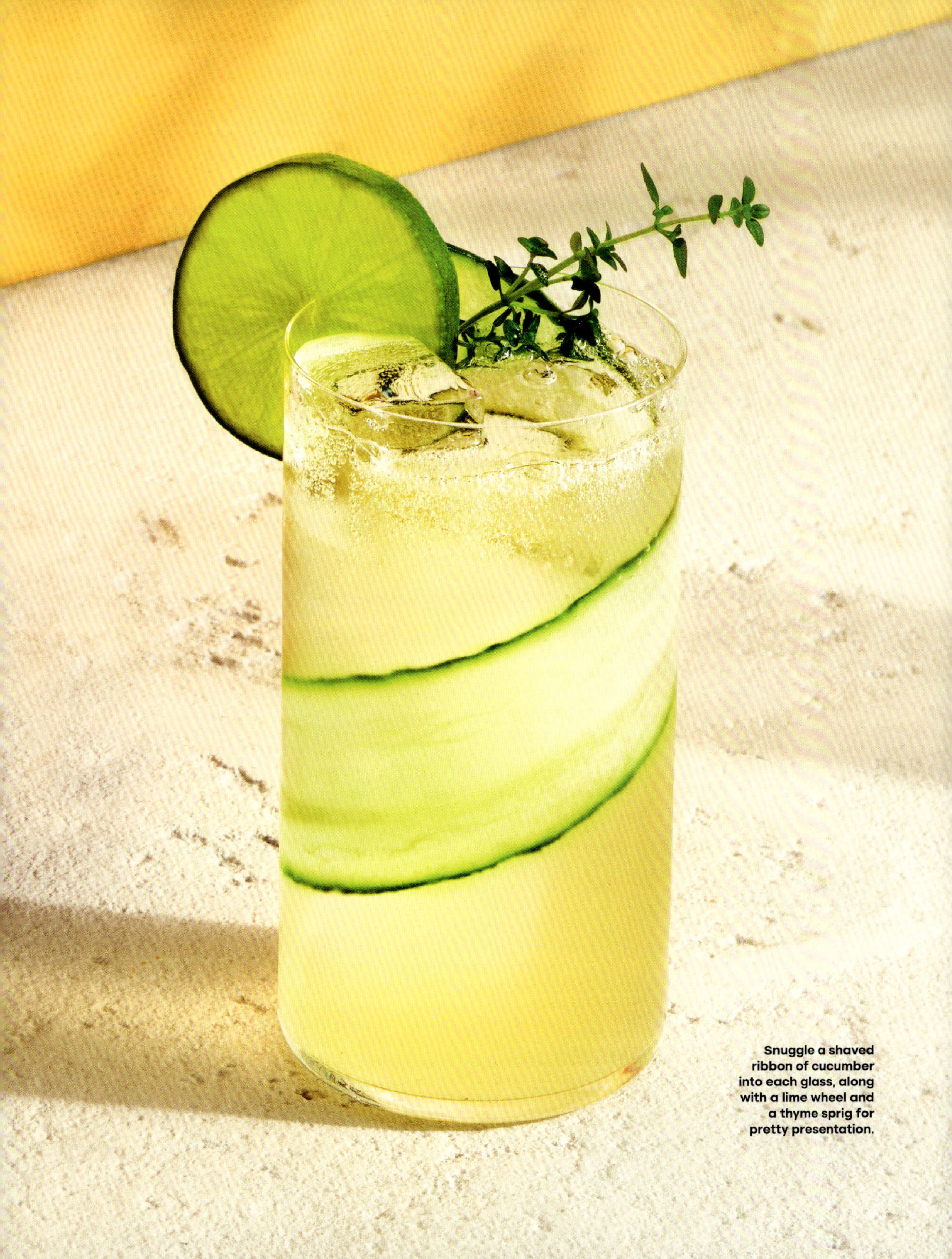

Snuggle a shaved ribbon of cucumber into each glass, along with a lime wheel and a thyme sprig for pretty presentation.

LOW-SUGAR SIPPER!

Ginger Citrus Spritz

- **1¼** cups fresh grapefruit juice
- **½** cup fresh lemon juice, plus lemon twists for serving
- **1** 2-inch piece fresh ginger, peeled and thinly sliced
- **2** Tbsp pure maple syrup
- Pinch of cayenne pepper
- Ice, for serving
- **1** liter grapefruit seltzer, chilled

1. In small saucepan, combine both juices, ginger, maple syrup, and cayenne. Bring to a gentle simmer, remove from heat, and let steep for 10 minutes.

2. Strain juice mixture through a fine-mesh sieve into a jar, cover, and refrigerate until cold, about 1 hour.

3. For each serving, pour ¼ cup juice mixture into ice-filled glass, top with scant ¾ cup grapefruit seltzer. Garnish with lemon twist.

Serves 6. Per serving: About 42 cal, 0 g fat (0 g sat), 0 mg chol, 2 mg sodium, 11 g carb, 0 g fiber, 9.5 g sugar (4 g added sugar), 0 g pro

GOOD-FOR-YOU INGREDIENTS This sunny-looking sip has health benefits, too. **Ginger** helps tame bloat and cramps, while **grapefruit** can give your skin a glow with vitamin C and antioxidants.

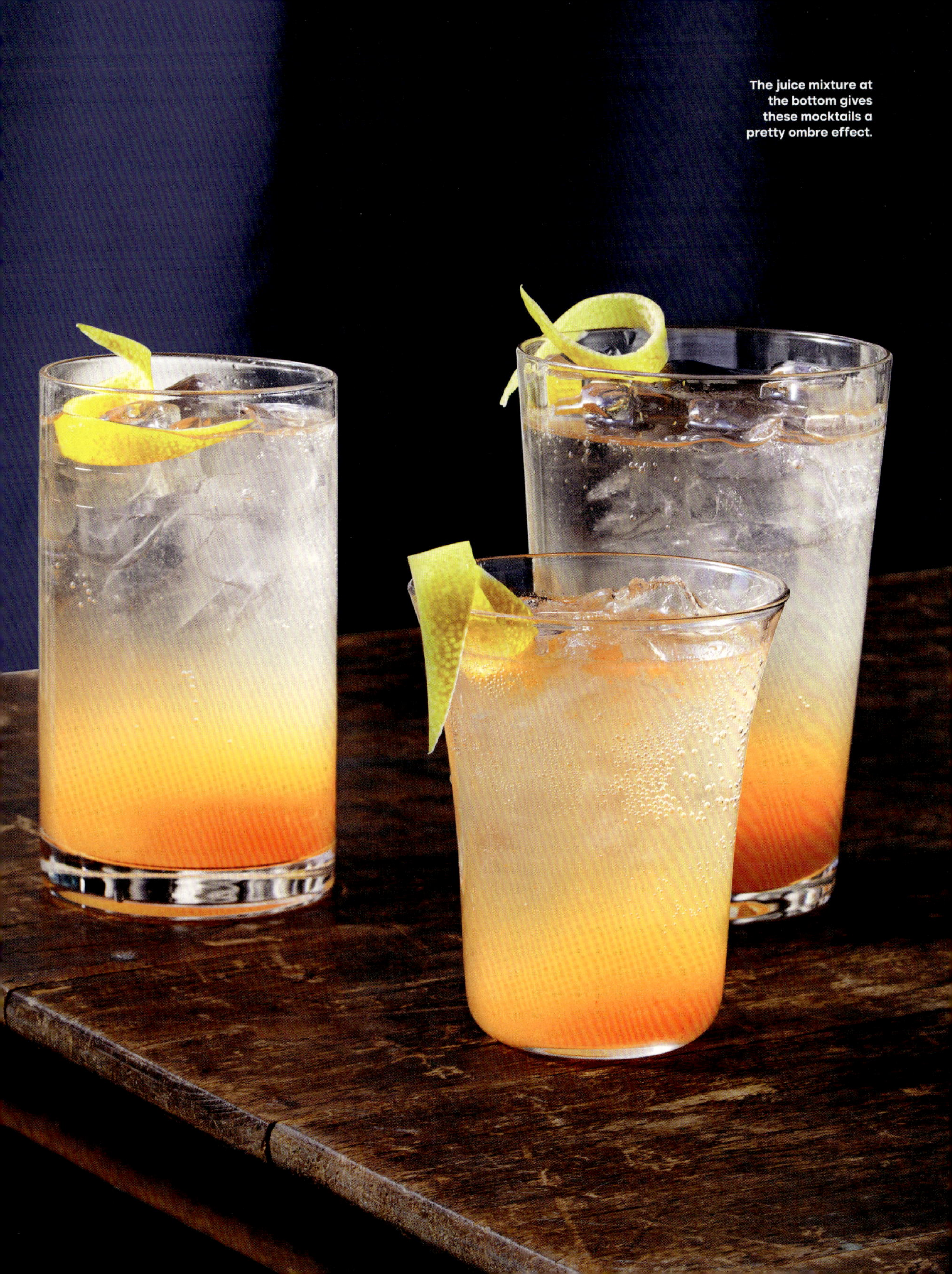

The juice mixture at the bottom gives these mocktails a pretty ombre effect.

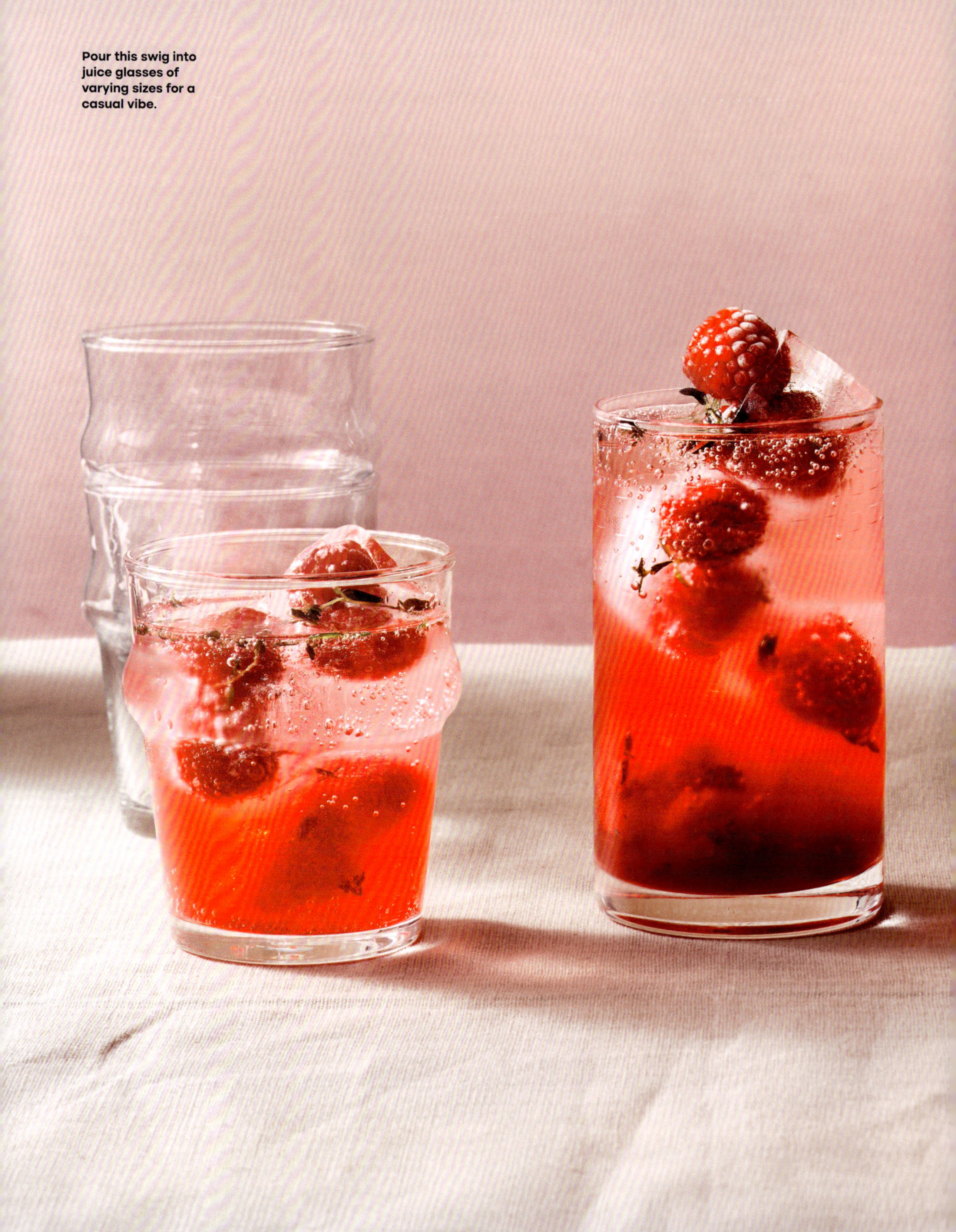

Pour this swig into juice glasses of varying sizes for a casual vibe.

Raspberry Hibiscus Mocktail

- **16** thyme sprigs, divided
- **2** pints fresh raspberries
- **2** hibiscus tea bags
- **1** cup frozen raspberries
- **½** cup sugar
- **1** Tbsp lemon zest plus 2 Tbsp lemon juice, divided
- **4½** cups sparkling water, chilled

1. Pick leaves from 6 thyme sprigs. Divide fresh raspberries and thyme leaves between 2 ice cube trays. Fill each tray three-quarters full with water and freeze until solid, at least 4 hours.

2. Meanwhile, in small saucepan, bring 1 cup water to a boil. Remove from heat, add tea bags, and let steep for 10 minutes. Remove tea bags and discard.

3. Measure out ½ cup tea, set aside the remainder, and return to the same saucepan. Add frozen raspberries, sugar, lemon zest, and remaining 10 thyme sprigs and bring to a boil. Simmer, stirring occasionally, for 5 minutes. Remove from heat and let sit for 10 minutes.

4. Strain raspberry-hibiscus syrup through a fine-mesh sieve into jar, pressing down on solids; discard solids. Cover and refrigerate until ice cubes are ready.

5. For each serving, in glass, stir 2 Tbsp raspberry-hibiscus syrup and 1 tsp lemon juice. Fill with raspberry-thyme ice cubes and gently stir in about 6 oz sparkling water.

Serves 6. Per serving: About 85 cal, 0 g fat, (0 g sat fat), 0 mg chol, 40 mg sodium, 20 g carb, 1 g fiber, 18 g sugar, (17 g added sugar), 0 g pro

PRO TIP Pop raspberries and thyme leaves into your ice cube trays for a pretty flourish,

Watermelon Mint Spritz

- **4** oz sparkling water
- **1½** oz watermelon juice
- **¾** oz lime juice
- **¾** oz Simple Syrup (recipe below)
- Ice, for shaking and serving
- **6** mint leaves, for serving

1 Pour sparkling water into 12- to 16-oz glass, such as a tulip glass.

2 In shaker, combine juices and Simple Syrup. Add a few ice cubes and shake 5 to 10 seconds. Strain over the sparkling water, then add ice and garnish with mint.

Serves 1. Per serving: About 68 cal, 0 g fat, (0 g sat fat), 0 mg chol, 26 mg sodium, 18 g carb, 0 g fiber, 16 g sugar, (12.5 g added sugar), 0 g pro

Simple Syrup

COMBINE 1 cup sugar and 1 cup water in small saucepan over medium heat. Stir occasionally to warm the mixture until the sugar dissolves (no need to boil). **REMOVE** mixture from the heat and let cool. **POUR** mixture into a jar or bottle. Simple Syrup will keep in the fridge for up to a month.

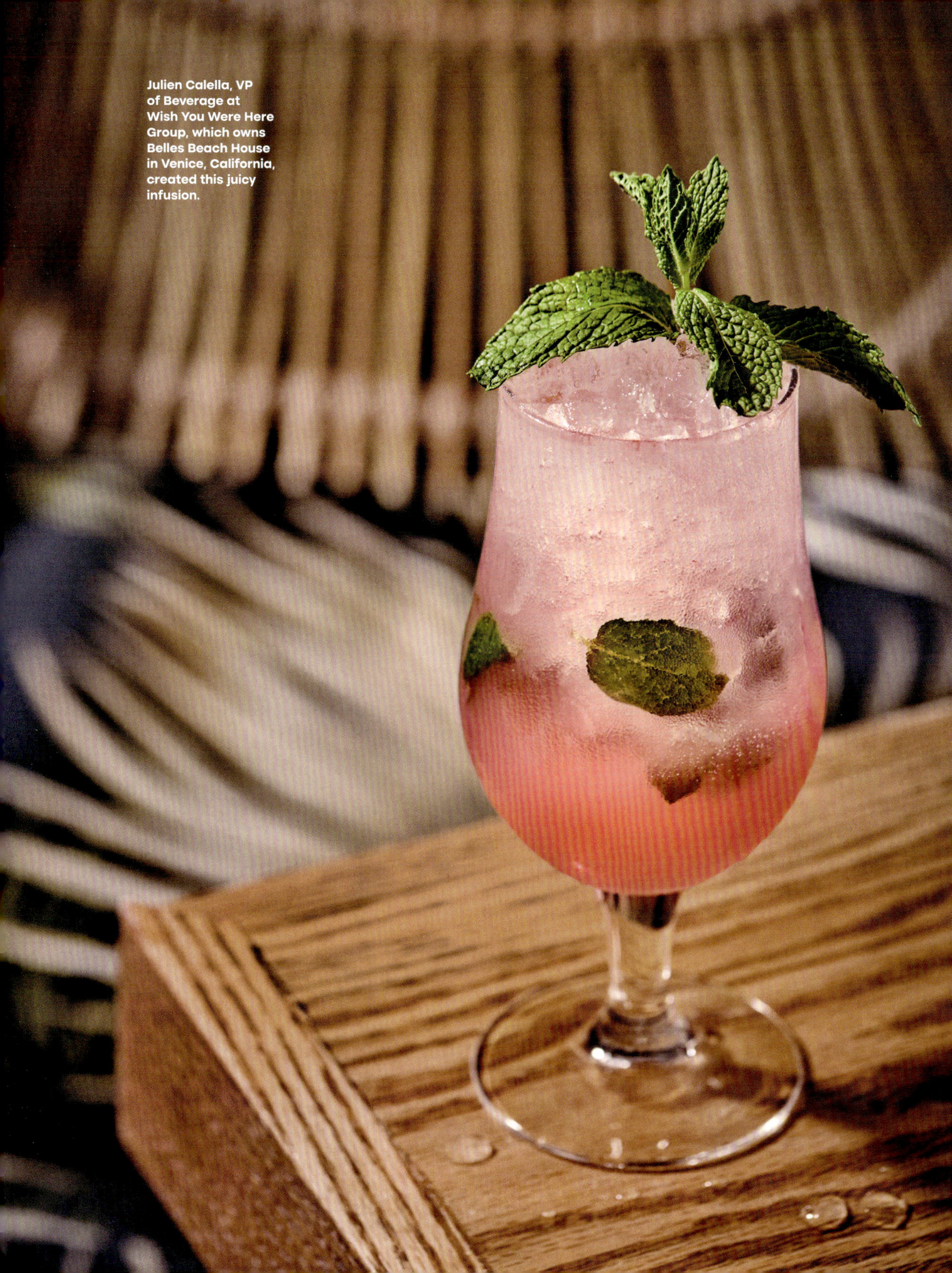

Julien Calella, VP of Beverage at Wish You Were Here Group, which owns Belles Beach House in Venice, California, created this juicy infusion.

At Lil Deb's Oasis, an LGBTQ+ friendly bar, restaurant, and art venue in Hudson, New York, locals sip the Grill Seeker with "tropical comfort food" like plantains, fried fish, and chicken with achiote rub, yogurt, and green sauce.

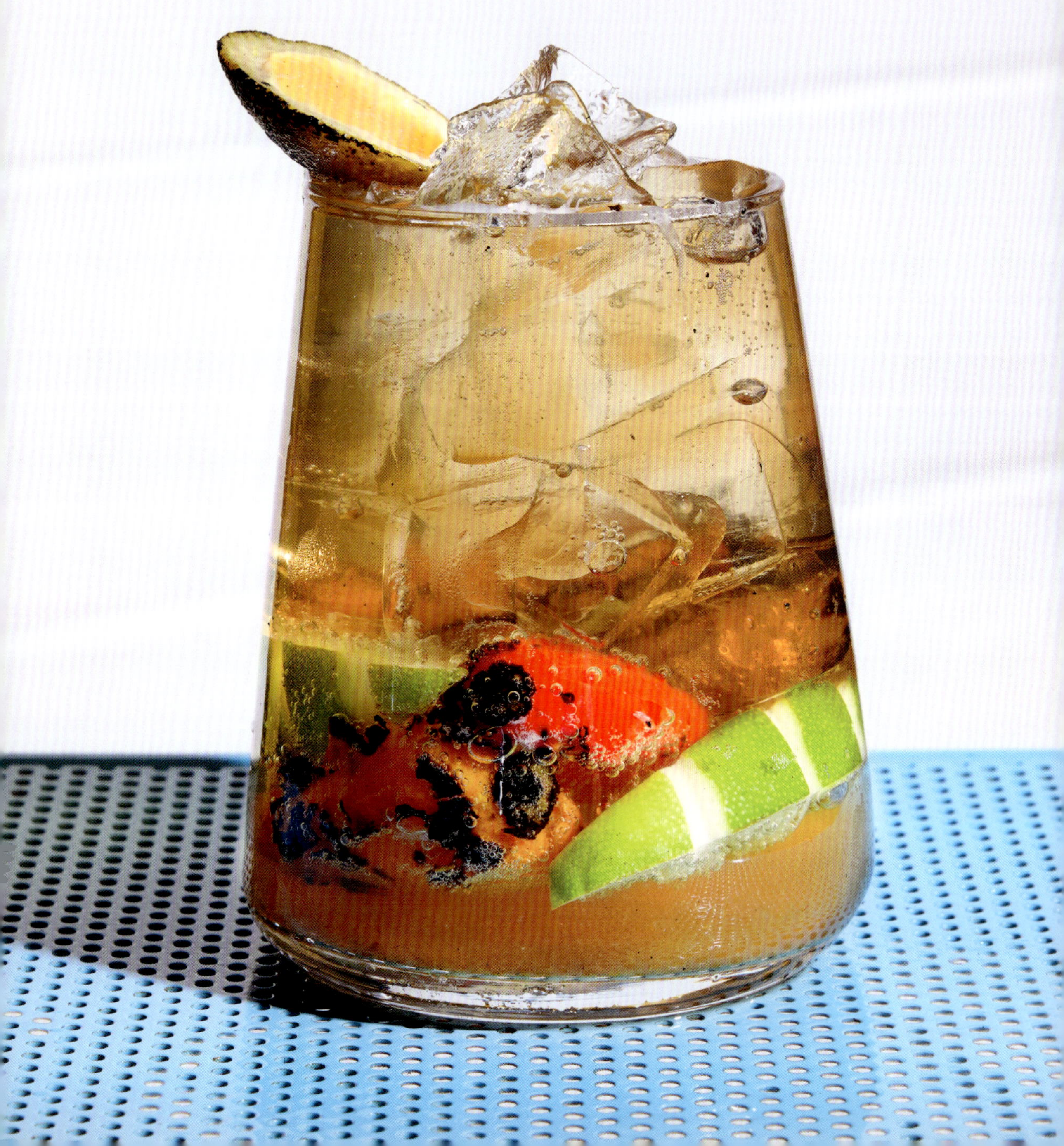

FLAVOR PROFILE This floral-accented sipper is both balanced and effervescent.

Grill Seeker

- **2–3** thin slices grilled peppers (red, yellow, or shishito all work well)
- **1–2** wedges grilled citrus such as lemon, lime, orange, or grapefruit—mix it up!
- **¾** oz Yerba Mate Simple Syrup (recipe below)
- Ice, for serving
- **3–4** oz soda water, chilled

1. In glass, muddle the peppers, citrus wedges, and Yerba Mate Simple Syrup.
2. Add ice, top with soda water and give it all a good stir with a swizzle stick or bar spoon.

Serves 1. Per serving: About 63 cal, 0.6 g fat, (0.15 g sat fat), 0.4 mg chol, 51 mg sodium, 15 g carb, 0.8 g fiber, 14 g sugar, (12.6 g added sugar), 0.35 g pro

INGREDIENT EXPLAINER

Yerba mate is a caffeinated herbal tea made from the stems and leaves of the yerba mate plant; it's popular in South America. Find it at Amazon, Target, and select grocery stores.

Yerba Mate Simple Syrup

STEEP 2 to 3 Tbsp loose yerba mate or 2 yerba mate tea bags in 1 cup hot (not boiling) water (about 175°F) for 5 to 7 minutes. **LET** tea cool a bit, then strain it into a heat-proof jar. **STIR** in 1 cup sugar to dissolve. **CHILL** before use. You can also add a splash of this syrup to sparkling water, along with a squeeze of lemon or lime, for a refreshing beverage.

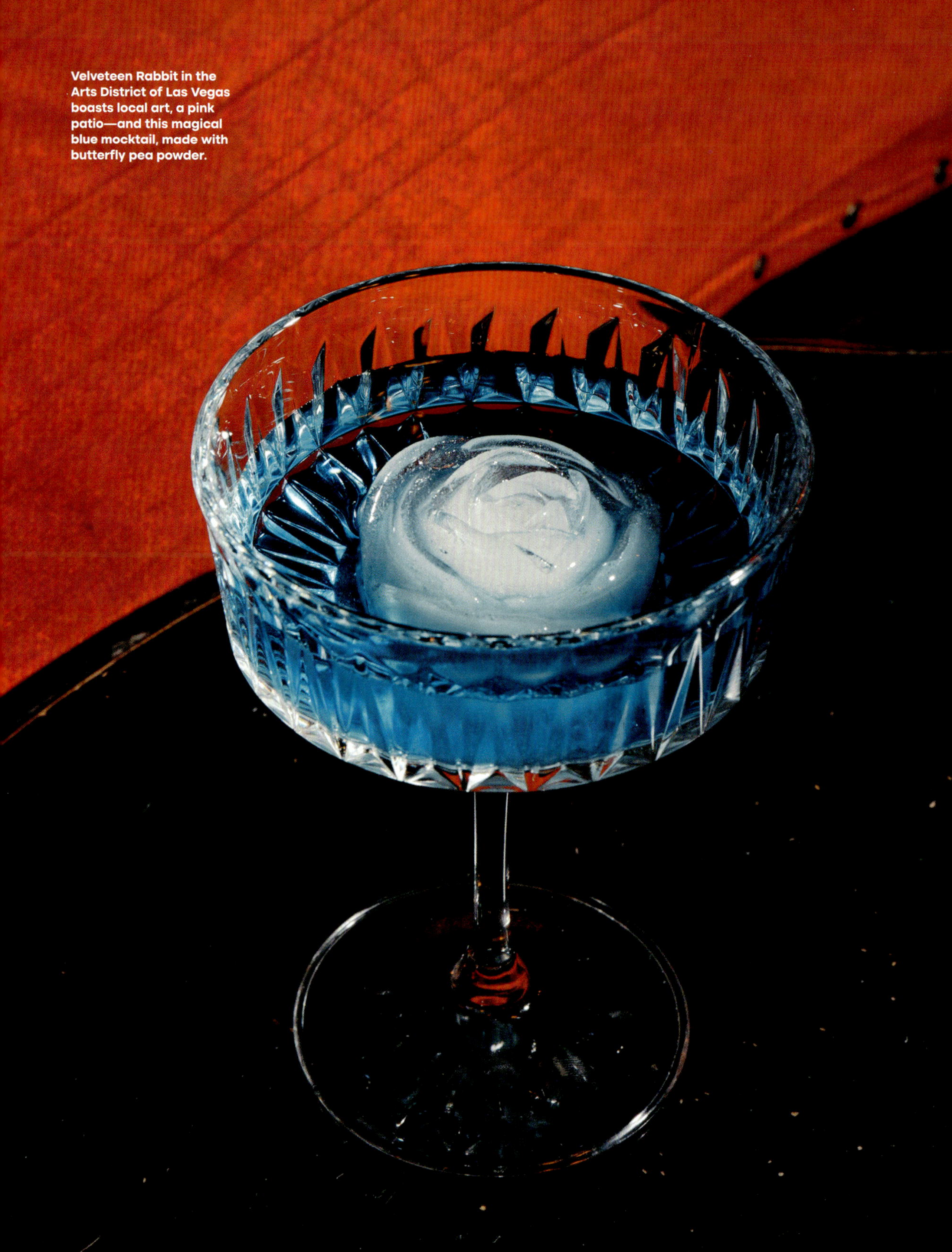

Velveteen Rabbit in the Arts District of Las Vegas boasts local art, a pink patio—and this magical blue mocktail, made with butterfly pea powder.

Love-in-Idleness

- **1** oz non-alcoholic gin (such as Lyre's)
- **½** oz lemon juice
- **½** oz lemongrass syrup (such as Bluestem Botanicals)
- **2¼** oz Butterfly Honeysuckle Tea, (recipe below)
- **1** oz Mediterranean tonic (such as Fever-Tree)
- Ice, for shaking
- Large ice cube, for serving

1. In shaker with ice, combine gin, lemon juice, and lemongrass syrup and shake until shaker is frosty.

2. Strain into a coupe glass with a single large ice cube. Add Butterfly Honeysuckle Tea and tonic, stir, and serve.

Serves 1. Per serving: 178 cal, 1 g fat, (0.01 g sat fat), 0 mg chol, 8 mg sodium, 34.6 g carb, 0.05 g fiber, 19.6 g sugar, (10.6 g added sugar), 7.6 g pro

INGREDIENT EXPLAINER

This bev gets its blue hue from **butterfly pea powder**, made from the butterfly pea plant, a vine native to Southeast Asia. You can also try this powder frothed in warm "Blue Moon" milk with maple syrup, cinnamon, cardamom, and nutmeg before bed. Both butterfly pea powder and **dried honeysuckle blossoms** can be found on Amazon. **Mediterranean tonic** is more aromatic than standard tonic, with hints of herbs and citrus.

Butterfly Honeysuckle Tea

BOIL 4½ cups water. **POUR** boiling water over a mix of 10g butterfly pea powder and 7½ g loose dried honeysuckle blossoms in saucepan or large heat-proof measuring cup. **STRAIN** through fine-mesh sieve into a pitcher. **ADD** 1 liter cold water and chill before using.

Ruby Scent

- **4** basil leaves, plus more for serving
- **3/4** oz fresh lime juice
- **1/2** oz orgeat syrup
- **1 1/3** oz puree of strawberries and raspberries
- **1 3/4** oz cranberry juice
- Ice, for shaking and serving
- Sparkling water, chilled, for topping off
- Fresh berries, for serving

1 In shaker, gently muddle 4 basil leaves with lime juice and orgeat syrup.

2 Add berry puree, cranberry juice, and ice. Shake until shaker is frosty.

3 Strain into an ice-filled glass. Top with sparkling water. Garnish with basil and a few fresh berries.

Serves 1. Per serving: About 80 cal, 0 g fat, (0 g sat fat), 0 mg chol, 22 mg sodium, 20 g carb, 1 g fiber, 16 g sugar, (8 g added sugar), 1 g pro

INGREDIENT EXPLAINER

Orgeat syrup is a regular in tiki drinks, imparting a creamy, nutty taste. It's made from almonds and orange flower water (and sometimes cinnamon, cloves, and vanilla). Try a drizzle over plums, peaches, or ice cream. Find orgeat syrup on Amazon or at a specialty store.

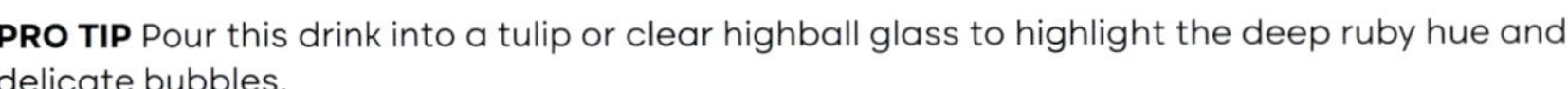

PRO TIP Pour this drink into a tulip or clear highball glass to highlight the deep ruby hue and delicate bubbles.

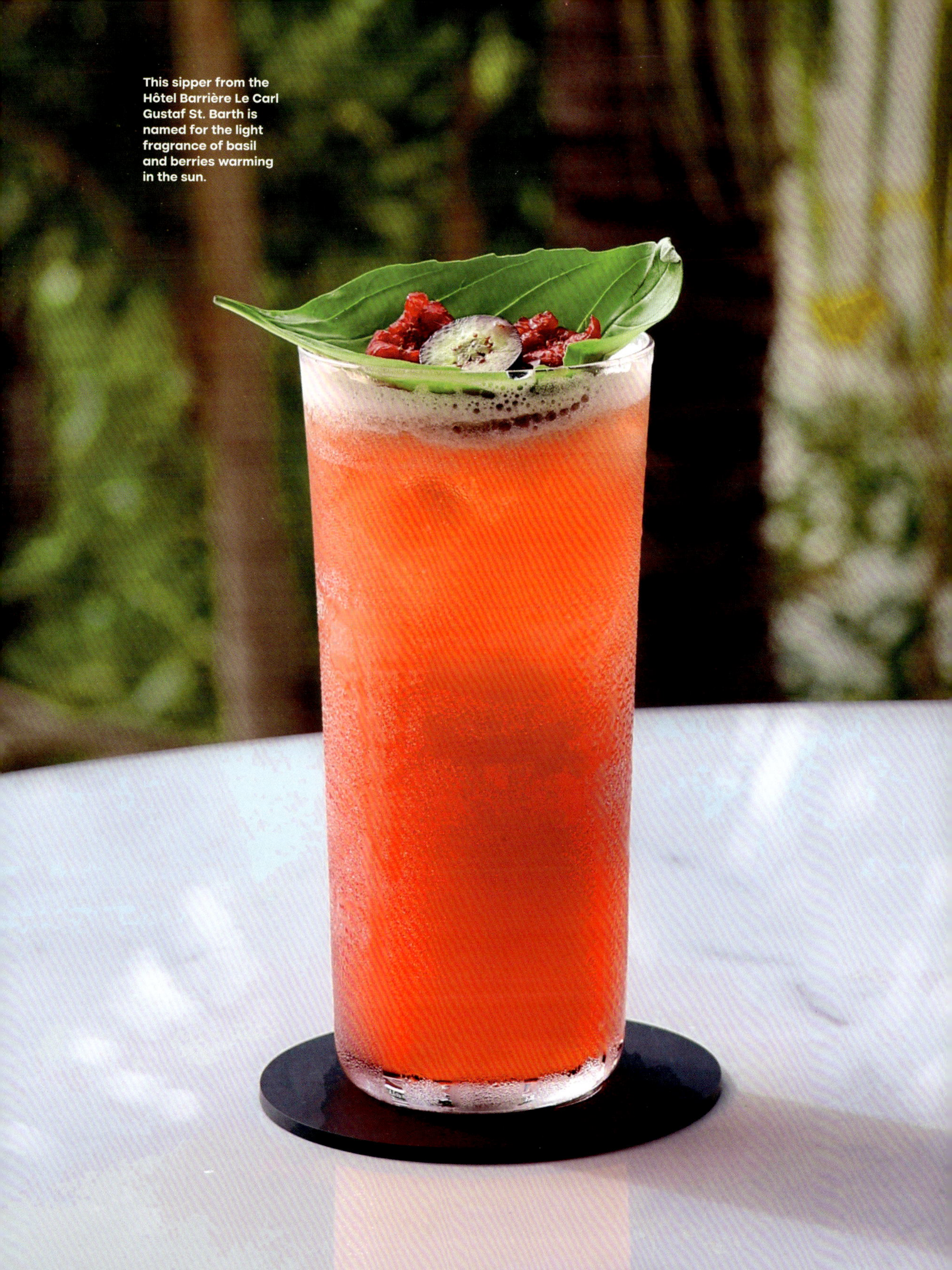

This sipper from the Hôtel Barrière Le Carl Gustaf St. Barth is named for the light fragrance of basil and berries warming in the sun.

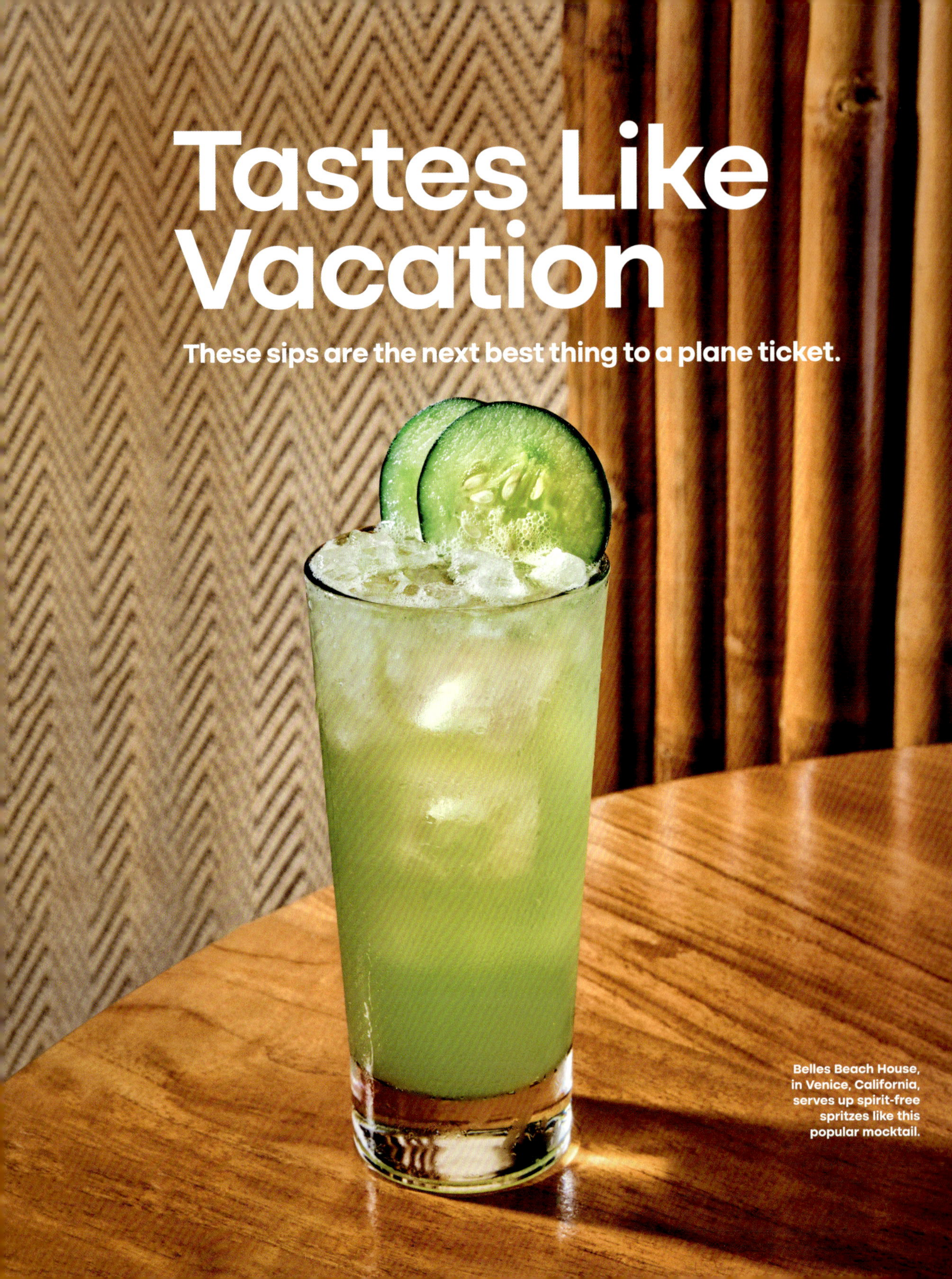

Tastes Like Vacation

These sips are the next best thing to a plane ticket.

Belles Beach House, in Venice, California, serves up spirit-free spritzes like this popular mocktail.

FLAVOR PROFILE This drink is bright, citrusy, and as refreshing as an island breeze.

Palm Reader

- **2** oz soda water, chilled
- **1½** oz Aplós Ease or similar botanical non-alcoholic spirit (like Ghia or The Pathfinder)
- **¾** oz Yuzu Super Juice (such as Yuzuco) or yuzu or equal parts lemon and lime juice
- **¾** oz simple syrup (store-bought or use recipe, p. 56)
- Ice, for shaking and serving
- Cucumber slices and basil leaves, for serving

1. Fill a highball glass with ice and add soda water.
2. In shaker with ice, add all ingredients (except cucumber and basil) and shake until shaker is frosty.
3. Strain mocktail into prepared highball glass. Garnish with cucumber slices and basil leaves.

Serves 1. Per serving: About 57 cal, 0 g fat, (0 g sat fat), 0 mg chol, 28 mg sodium, 14 g carb, 0 g fiber, 11 g sugar, (11 g added sugar), 0 g pro

INGREDIENT EXPLAINER

Yuzu is a complex, aromatic, Chinese citrus fruit about the size of a tangerine. You can find Yuzu Super Juice at Asian grocery stores and on Amazon. Try a splash in salad dressing, on seafood, or in a marinade.

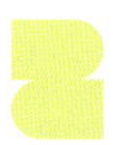

RAISE THE BAR Functional spirits feature ingredients with benefits beyond nutrition. **Aplós Ease** is a blend of citrus and herbal extracts, plus lion's mane and magnesium, which promote calm.

LOW-SUGAR SIPPER!

Lemongrass Mint Nojito

- **3** stalks lemongrass
- **6** green tea bags
- **2** Tbsp honey
- **6** sprigs mint, divided, plus more for serving
- Ice, for serving

1. Cut lemongrass stalks in half lengthwise, then smash with the back of a knife.

2. Place in large saucepan, add 6 cups water, and bring to a boil. Reduce heat and simmer 5 minutes.

3. Remove from heat, add tea bags and honey, and let steep 5 minutes; let cool.

4. Strain into pitcher. Stir in 2 cups cold water. Serve in rocks glasses over ice with mint.

Serves 6. Per serving: About 36 cal, 0 g fat (0 g sat), 0 mg chol, 9 mg sodium, 9 g carb, 0 g fiber, 8.5 g sugar (8 g added sugar), 1 g pro

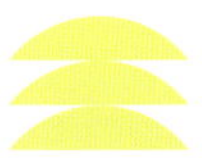

LIFE AFTER ALCOHOL: "I dated myself"

When Tawny first got sober, dating was off the table—but self-discovery was very much on. "Early sobriety can be a really vulnerable time," she says. "Not only was I learning to live without alcohol, but I had to sit with—and make sense of—the feelings I'd been avoiding for years." To fill that space, she started doing all the things she used to dream about. "I took writing courses, studied Spanish, and even signed up for an improv class. I called it my era of dating myself."

Lemongrass and mint are a dreamy combo in this iced tea cooler. The mint lends mojito vibes without the alcohol.

LOW-SUGAR SIPPER!

Coconut Fizz

- **2** green tea bags
- **¼** cup coconut milk
- **2** Tbsp fresh lime juice
- **½** cup coconut seltzer
- Ice, for serving
- Matcha powder, for serving

1. Pour ¼ cup boiling water over tea bags and let steep for 5 minutes; discard tea bags and let cool.
2. In pitcher, stir together tea, coconut milk, and lime juice.
3. Divide between 2 glasses filled with ice and top with seltzer. Dust with matcha powder.

Serves 2. Per serving: About 117 cal, 12 g fat (10.5 g sat), 0 mg chol, 21 mg sodium, 3 g carb, 0 g fiber, 0.5 g sugar (0 g added sugar), 2 g pro

PREP AHEAD Double or triple the batch of concentrated tea and keep it in the fridge so you can quickly make this mocktail when friends are over.

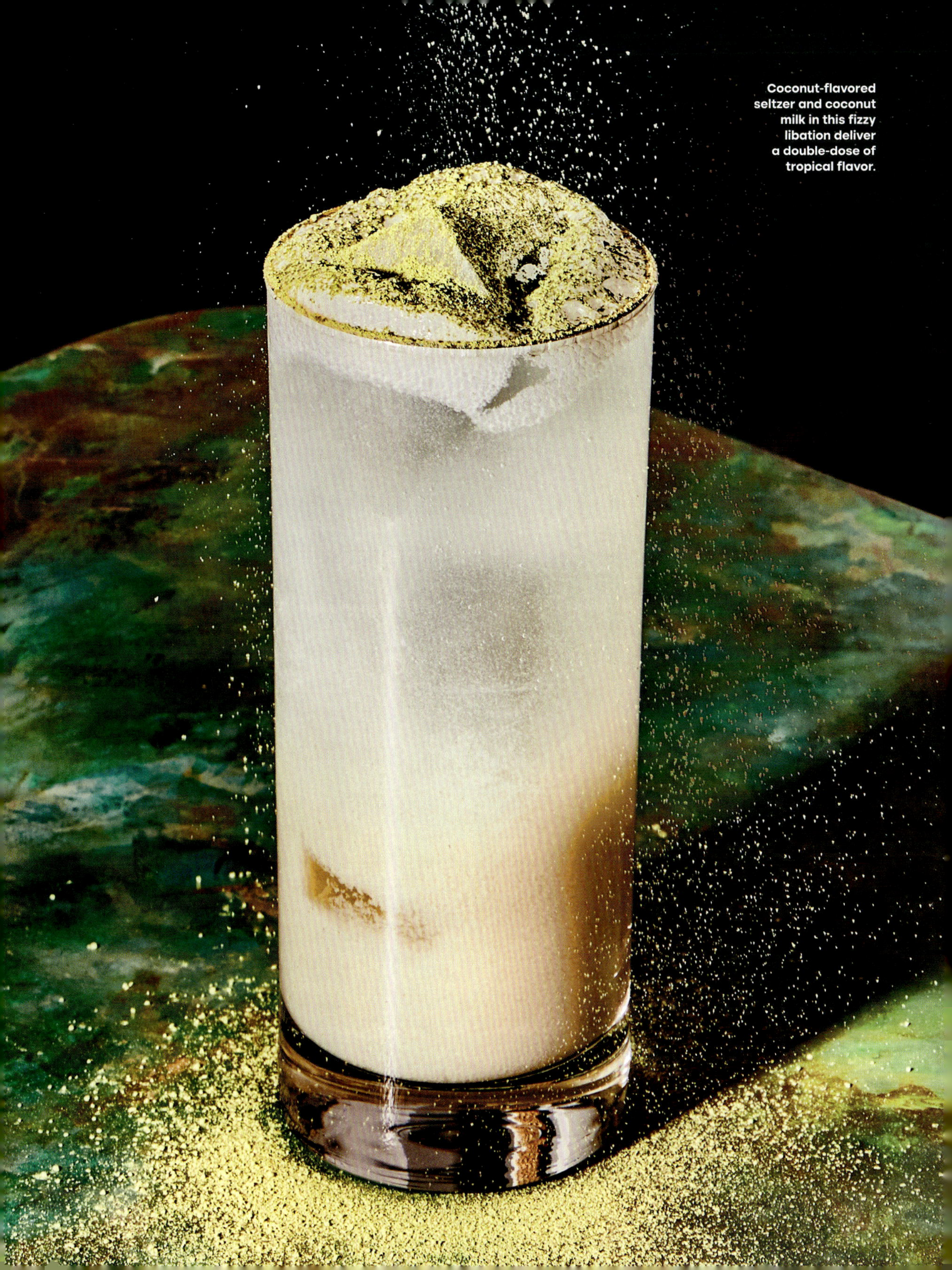

Coconut-flavored seltzer and coconut milk in this fizzy libation deliver a double-dose of tropical flavor.

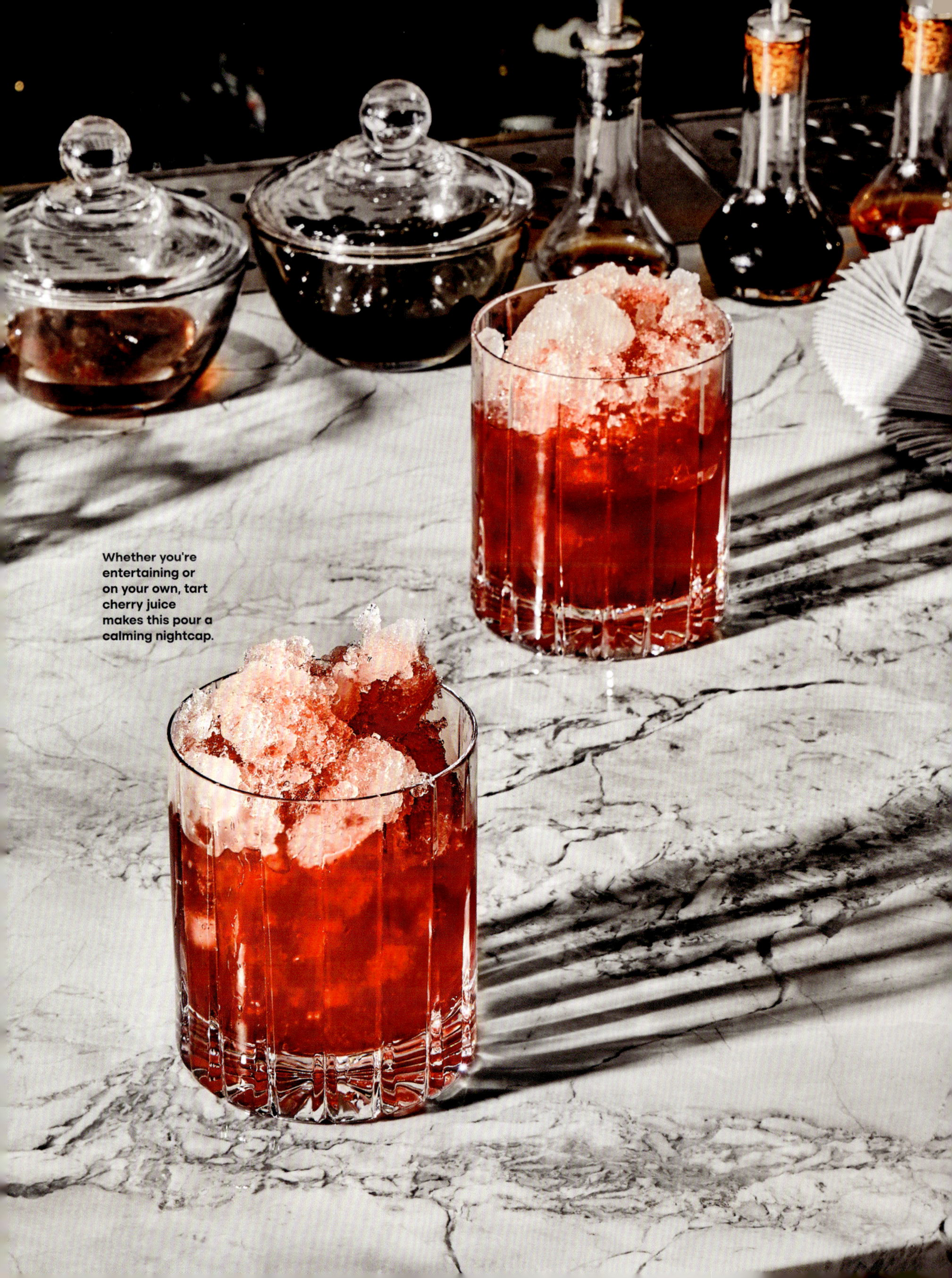

Whether you're entertaining or on your own, tart cherry juice makes this pour a calming nightcap.

Cherry Crush

- **4** whole cloves
- **1** whole star anise
- **1** 1-inch piece fresh ginger, sliced
- **1** Tbsp agave
- **4** cups tart cherry juice, chilled
- Ice, for serving
- **2** 12-oz cans berry-flavored prebiotic soda (such as Poppi in Raspberry Rose), chilled

1. In small saucepan, combine cloves, star anise, ginger, agave, and ½ cup water. Bring to a simmer, then simmer for 3 minutes. Let cool completely.

2. Strain syrup into pitcher and stir in cherry juice.

3. Divide mixture among ice-filled old-fashioned glasses, then top each glass with ½ cup prebiotic soda.

Serves 6. Per serving: About 104 cal, 0 g fat (0 g sat), 0 mg chol, 15 mg sodium, 26 g carb, 1 g fiber, 20 g sugar (3.5 g added sugar), 0 g pro

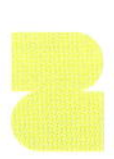

GOOD-FOR-YOU INGREDIENT Tart **cherry juice** contains melatonin and tryptophan for a better night's sleep. **Prebiotic soda** has beneficial bacteria to support gut health.

FLAVOR PROFILE This bold pitcher drink delivers citrusy refreshment, with a touch of complexity from chamomile and cucumber.

Blue Wave

- **24** chamomile tea bags
- **¾** cup sugar
- **1–2** tsp blue spirulina powder
- **1** English cucumber
- **6** strips lime zest plus 6 lime wheels, for serving
- **¾** cup fresh lemon juice, divided
- **¾** cup fresh lime juice, divided
- Ice, for shaking and serving
- **36** oz club soda, chilled
- **6** thyme sprigs, for serving

1. In medium saucepan, bring 3 cups water to a boil. Remove from heat. Add tea bags and sugar, and stir until sugar dissolves. Let steep for 10 minutes. Strain, squeezing tea bags, into liquid measuring cup; discard tea bags.

2. Whisk in spirulina powder. Let tea cool to room temperature, about 15 minutes.

3. Meanwhile, cut 12 round slices from cucumber and set aside.

4. In large shaker, muddle 2 strips lime zest and 4 cucumber slices with 2 oz cooled chamomile tea. Add ¼ cup lemon juice, ¼ cup lime juice. and 6 oz chamomile tea; fill shaker with ice and shake until shaker is frosty.

5. Strain through a coffee filter into a pitcher (to eliminate any blue specks). Repeat shaking and straining 2 more times.

6. Serve in glasses over ice, gently stir 6 oz club soda into each glass, then garnish with lime wheels and thyme sprigs.

Serves 6. Per serving: About 124 cal, 0 g fat, (0 g sat fat), 0 mg chol, 57 mg sodium, 32 g carb, 0 g fiber, 27 g sugar, (25 g added sugar), 1 g pro

PRO TIP For the brightest blue, use tea bags filled with whole rather than crushed chamomile flowers in this refreshing libation.

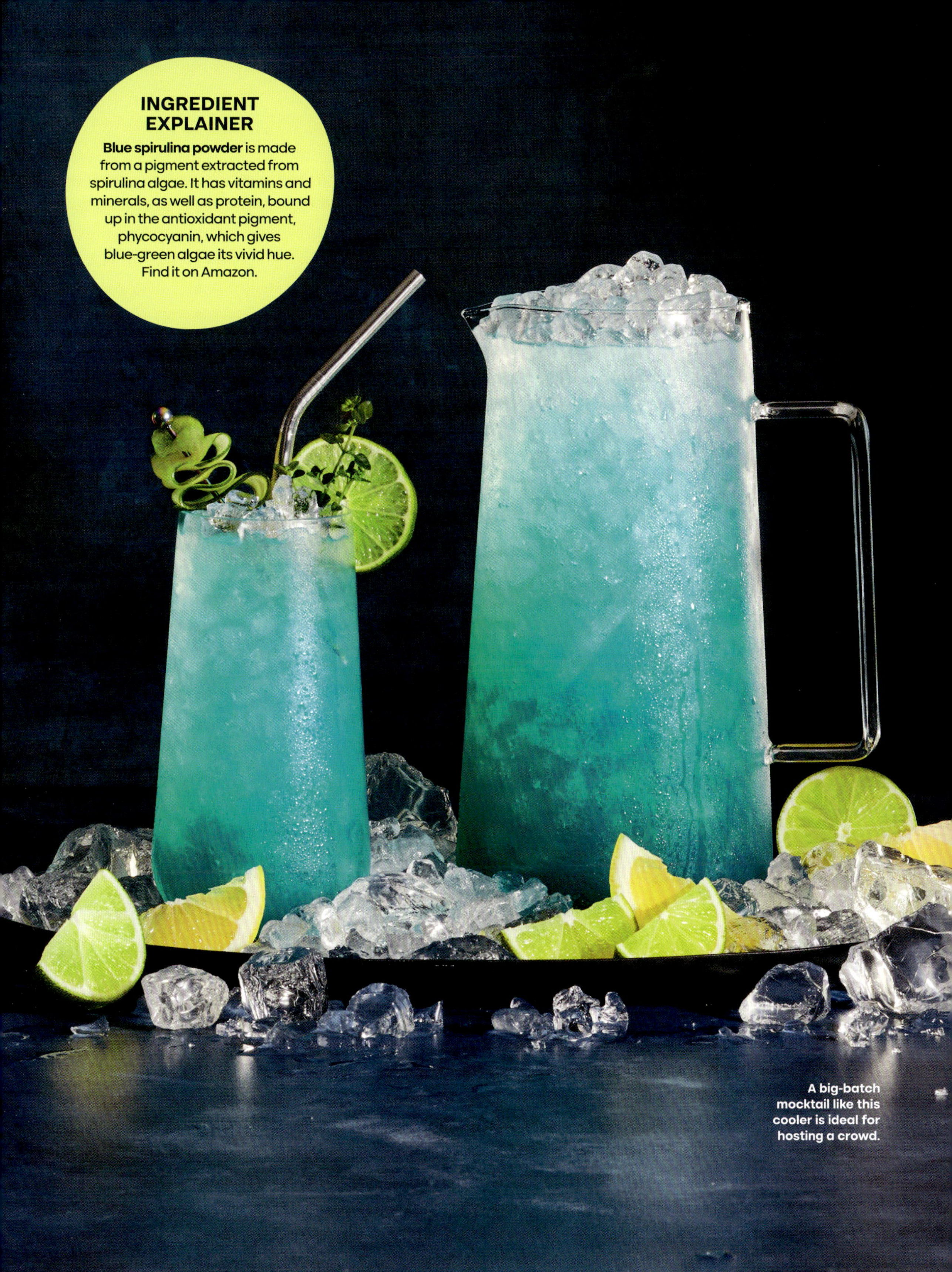

INGREDIENT EXPLAINER

Blue spirulina powder is made from a pigment extracted from spirulina algae. It has vitamins and minerals, as well as protein, bound up in the antioxidant pigment, phycocyanin, which gives blue-green algae its vivid hue. Find it on Amazon.

A big-batch mocktail like this cooler is ideal for hosting a crowd.

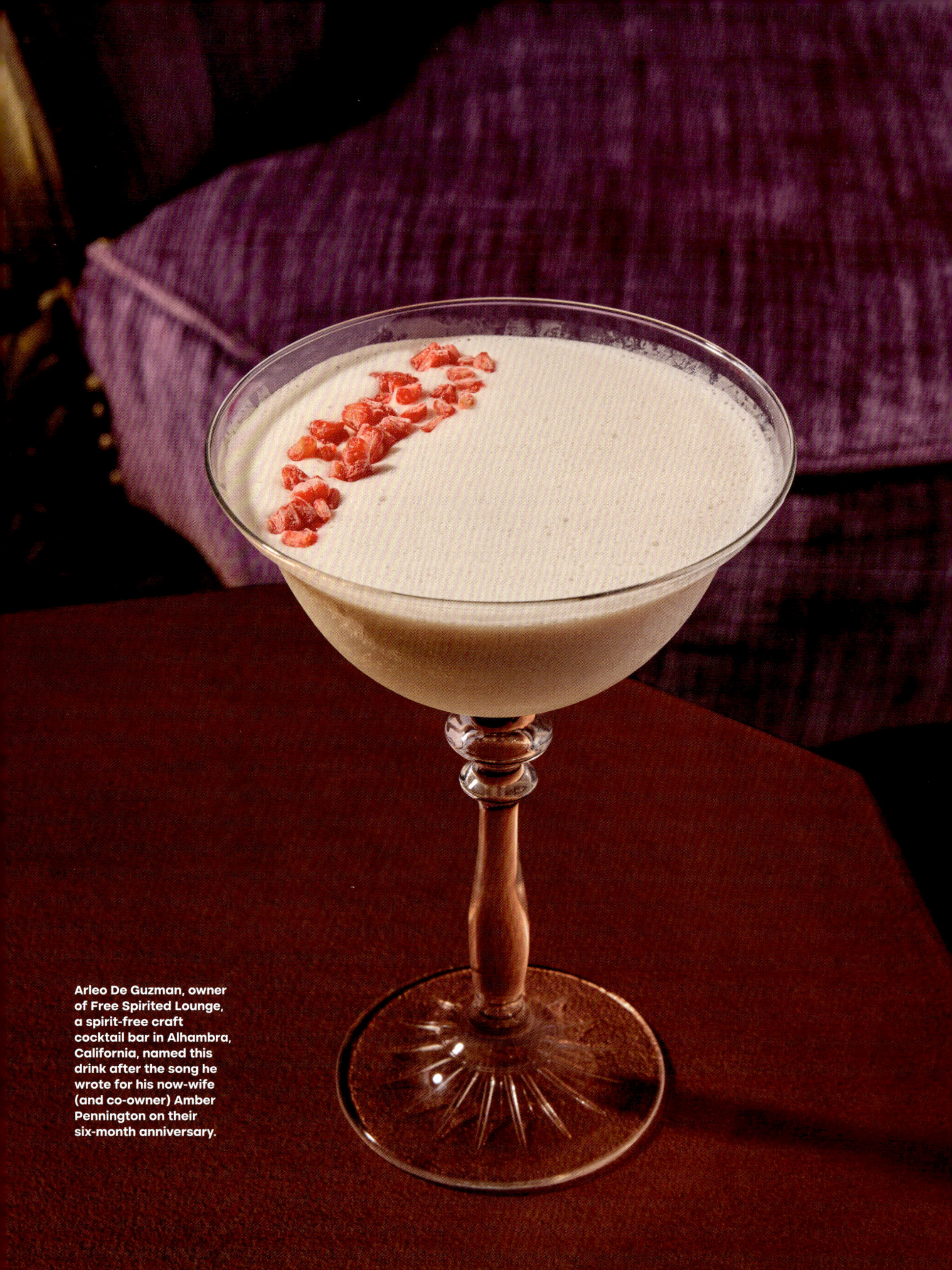

Arleo De Guzman, owner of Free Spirited Lounge, a spirit-free craft cocktail bar in Alhambra, California, named this drink after the song he wrote for his now-wife (and co-owner) Amber Pennington on their six-month anniversary.

FLAVOR PROFILE Piña colada lovers will go nuts for this tropical sipper, brightened by a touch of lemon juice.

Quarantine Heart

- **2 ½** oz pineapple juice
- **1** oz lemon juice
- **1** oz cream of coconut
- **½** oz Grenadine (recipe below or store-bought version made from pomegranate, such as Liquid Alchemist)
- Ice, for shaking and serving
- Pomegranate seeds, chopped, for serving, if desired

1. In shaker with ice, add all ingredients (except pomegranate seeds) and shake until shaker is frosty.

2. Strain mocktail into a large coupe or martini glass. Garnish with chopped pomegranate seeds, if desired.

Serves 1. Per serving: About 221 cal, 0 g fat, (0 g sat fat), 0 mg chol, 7 mg sodium, 53.5 g carb, 0 g fiber, 46 g sugar, (37 g added sugar), 0 g pro

Grenadine

COMBINE 1 cup pomegranate juice (fresh or bottled, 100% juice) and 1 cup sugar in small saucepan. Heat over medium, stirring until sugar fully dissolves, but don't let it boil. Once dissolved, remove from heat. **STIR** in 1 to 2 tsp rosewater. Start with 1 tsp, taste, and add more if desired. **LET COOL**, then pour into clean glass jar or bottle. **STORE** in the refrigerator for up to 1 month.

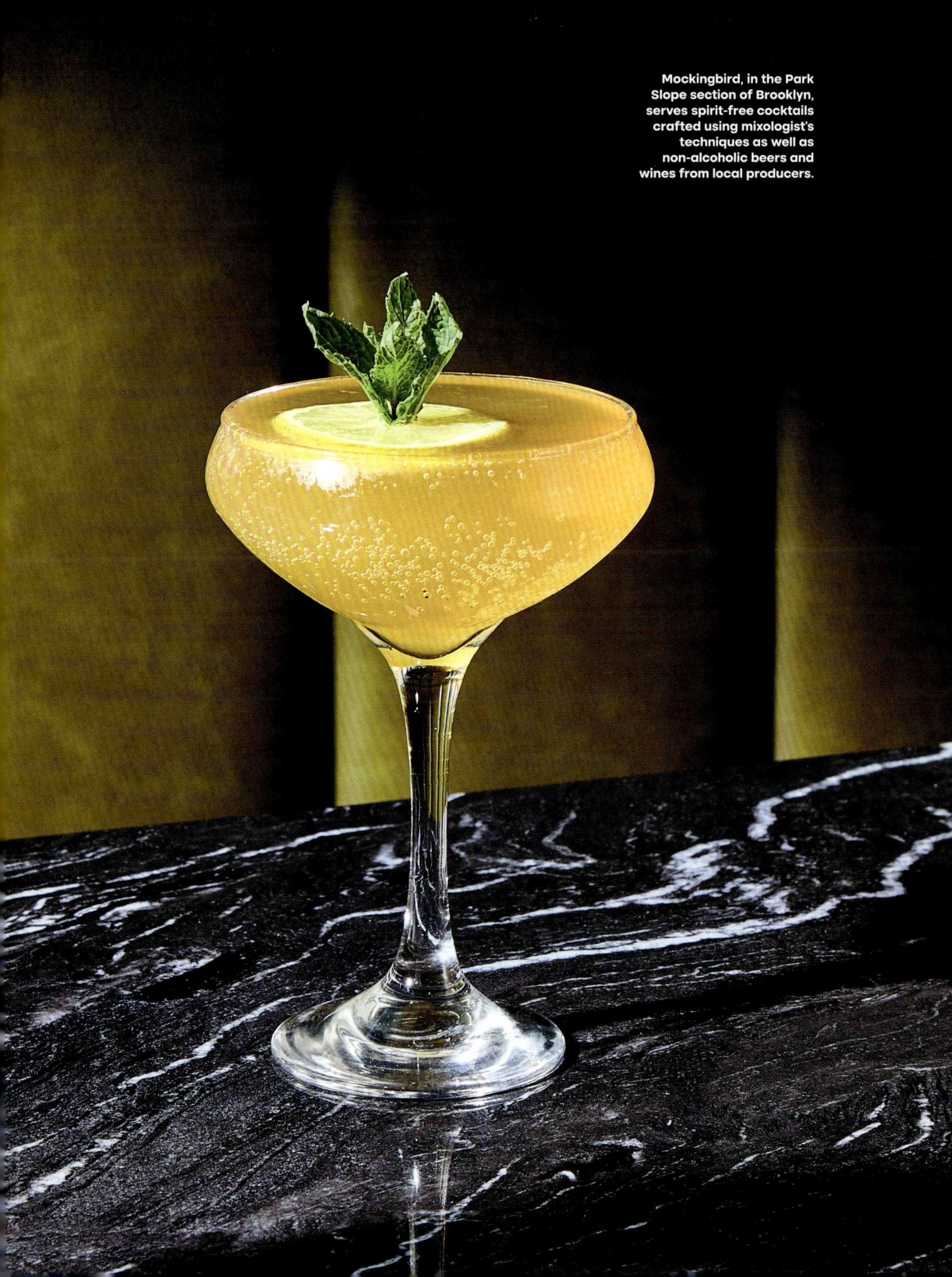

Mockingbird, in the Park Slope section of Brooklyn, serves spirit-free cocktails crafted using mixologist's techniques as well as non-alcoholic beers and wines from local producers.

Spring in Kyoto

- **2½** oz Hojicha Concentrate (recipe below)
- **1** oz Mint Syrup (recipe below)
- **¾** oz lemon juice
- Ice, for shaking
- Non-alcoholic sparkling wine (such as Moderato Blanc de Noir), for topping off
- Lemon wheel and mint sprig, for serving

1 In shaker with ice, shake Hojicha Concentrate, Mint Syrup, and lemon juice.

2 Strain into a chilled coupe glass and top with sparkling wine to fill the glass. Garnish with lemon wheel and mint.

Serves 1. Per serving: About 190 cal, 0 g fat, (0 g sat fat), 0 mg chol, 3 mg sodium, 45 g carb, 0 g fiber, 44 g sugar, (43 g added sugar), 1 g pro

INGREDIENT EXPLAINER

Hojicha is a mild green tea with hints of caramel and hazelnut. It's low in caffeine, so this mocktail won't mess with your sleep. Find hojicha at Whole Foods or on Amazon.

Hojicha Concentrate

COMBINE 3 tsp loose-leaf hojicha tea and 1 cup cold water in container and chill for 16 to 24 hours. **STRAIN** tea through fine-mesh sieve. **STORE** in fridge for up to 5 days. Add water to enjoy as iced tea.

Mint Syrup

COMBINE 1 cup water, 1 cup sugar, and 1 cup mint leaves in small saucepan. **BRING** to a boil, then reduce heat and simmer gently, for about 1 minute. **REMOVE** from heat and let steep for 30 minutes. **STRAIN** and store in fridge for up to 2 weeks. It's delish in iced tea.

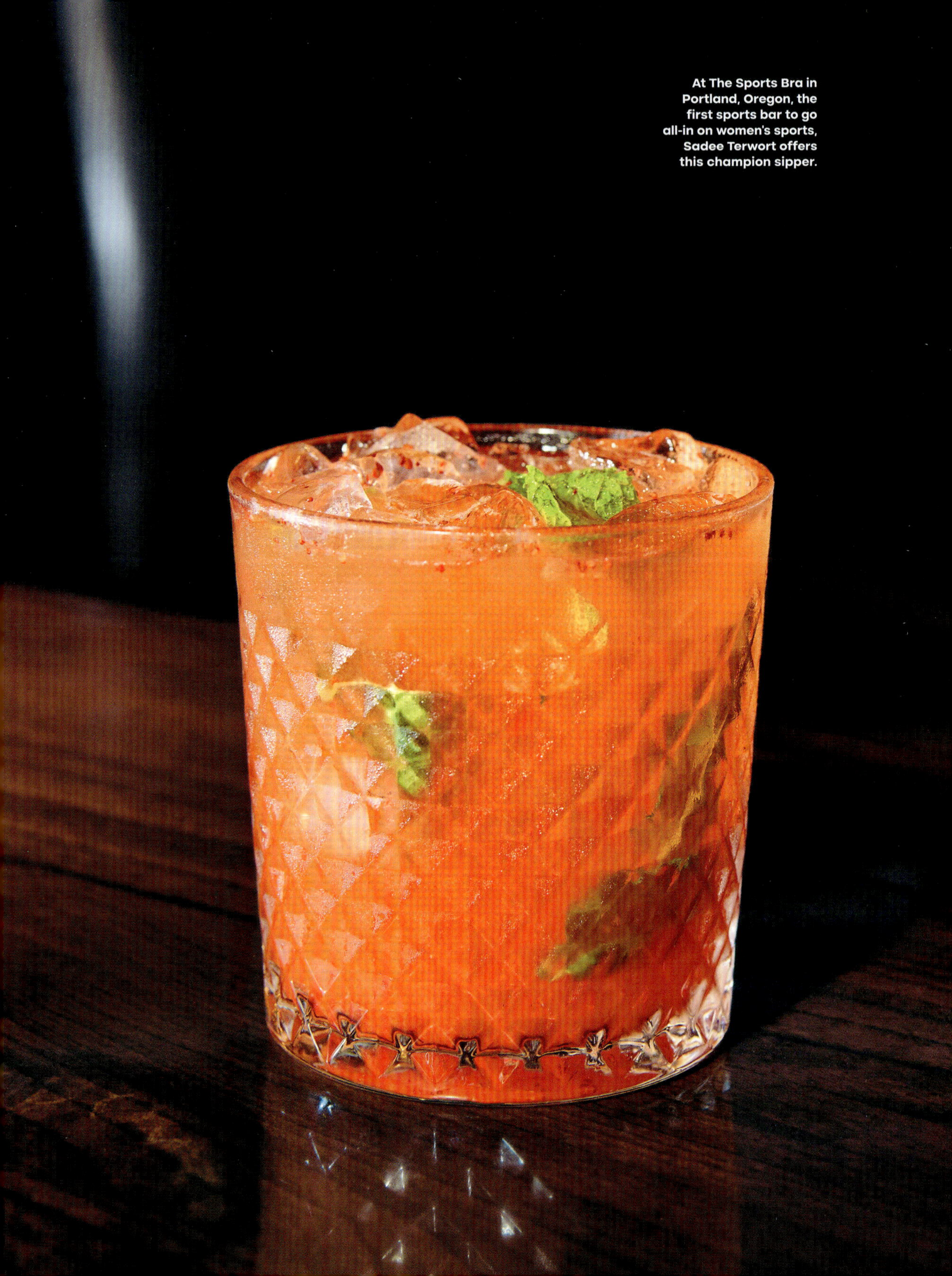

At The Sports Bra in Portland, Oregon, the first sports bar to go all-in on women's sports, Sadee Terwort offers this champion sipper.

The Strawskey Smash

- **4** oz non-alcoholic whiskey (such as Monday Zero Alcohol Whiskey)
- **2** oz pureed strawberries (about 4 large berries—just blend or mash them finely with a fork)
- **2** oz simple syrup (store-bought or use recipe, p. 56)
- **2** oz lemon juice
- **8** mint leaves
- Ice, for serving

In shaker, combine all ingredients and shake hard. Pour into 2 ice-filled glasses to serve.

Serves 2. Per serving: About 78 cal, 0 g fat, (0 g sat fat), 0 mg chol, 1.5 mg sodium, 20g carb, 7.5g fiber, 16.5 g sugar, (14.5 g added sugar), 1 g pro

PRO TIP For flavor, give the mint a quick muddle with a spoon before shaking.

Make a Pitcher

(SERVES 6–8)

COMBINE 12 oz non-alcoholic whiskey, 6 oz fresh strawberry puree, and 6 oz lemon juice in large pitcher. **SHAKE** 6 oz simple syrup and 24 mint leaves, torn or lightly muddled, in shaker and then add to the pitcher. **STIR** well to combine, then chill in the fridge for at least 30 minutes. When ready to serve, stir again, then pour into glasses filled with ice.

 **FLAVOR PROFILE** This fruit-forward, sour-style cocktail has a velvety mouthfeel.

Lemur's Tale

- 1½ oz non-alcoholic tequila (such as Free Spirits The Spirit of Tequila)
- 1 oz Baobab-Lychee Syrup (recipe below) or plain lychee syrup
- ¾ oz guava nectar
- ½ oz lime juice
- ¾ oz aquafaba (starchy liquid in a can of chickpeas)
- Ice, for shaking and serving
- Lychee and mint sprig on cocktail skewer, for serving

1. In shaker with ice, combine ingredients and shake until shaker is frosty.
2. Strain into coupe and garnish with skewered lychee and mint sprig.

Serves 6. Per serving: About 102 cal, 0 g fat, (0 g sat fat), 0 mg chol, 25 mg sodium, 26 g carb, 0.5 g fiber, 23 g sugar, (18 g added sugar), 0 g pro

INGREDIENT EXPLAINER

Baobab powder, made from the citrus-flavored fruit of the baobab tree, contains vitamin C, vitamin B6, niacin, iron, and potassium. You can find it on Amazon. **Aquafaba**, the liquid in a can of chickpeas, is a great emulsifier, adding froth to this cocktail. Roast the chickpeas for a crunchy snack to go with this swig.

Baobab-Lychee Syrup

COMBINE 2 cups sugar, 2 cups water, ½ tsp ground ginger, ½ tsp cardamom and 1 Tbsp baobab powder in medium saucepan. **BRING** to a simmer, stirring every few minutes, then remove from heat to cool for approximately 20 minutes. **ADD** 1 cup lychee syrup from a can of lychees. **POUR** mixture into a glass or bottle. Keep in the fridge for up to 1 week.

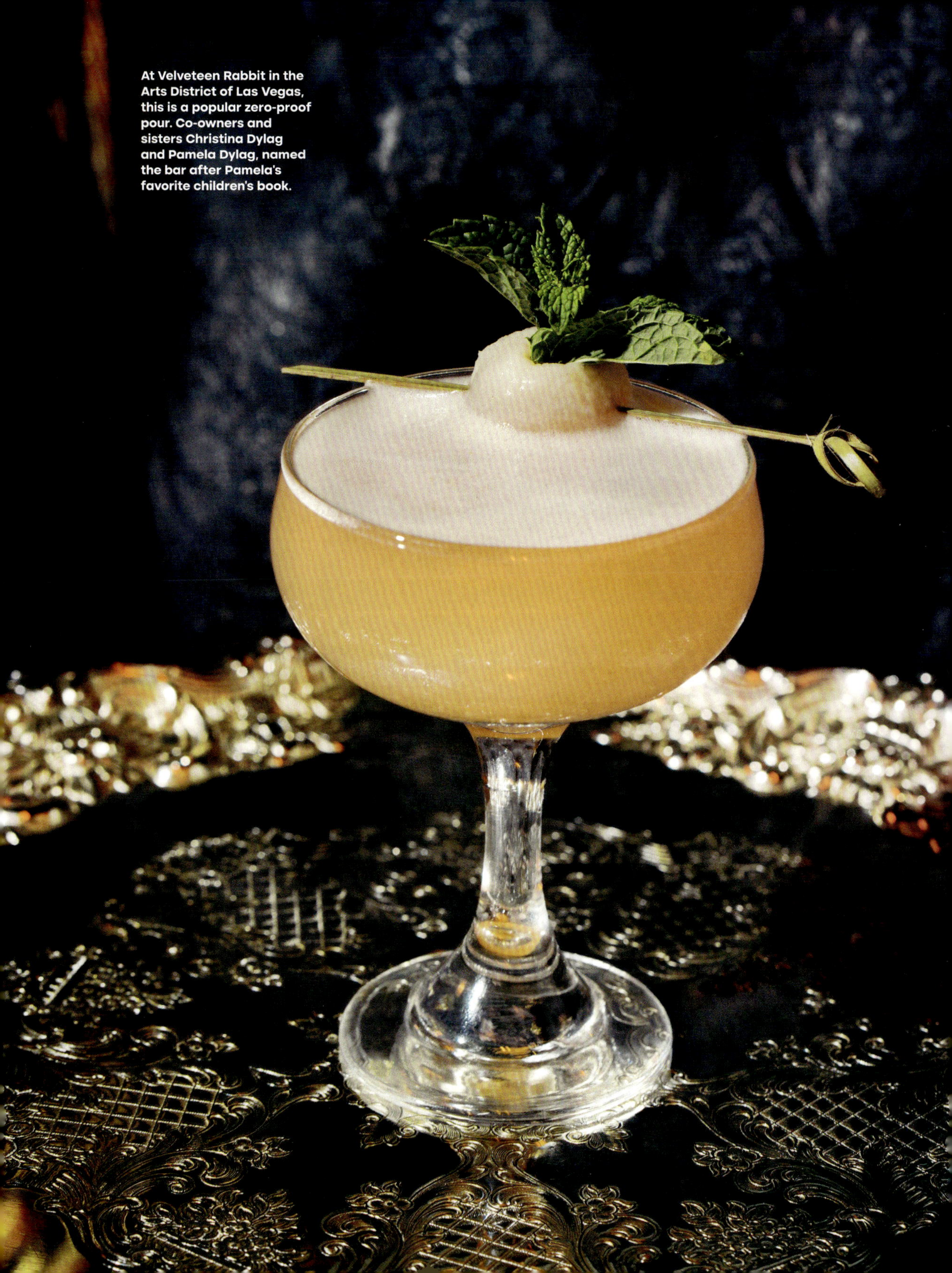

At Velveteen Rabbit in the Arts District of Las Vegas, this is a popular zero-proof pour. Co-owners and sisters Christina Dylag and Pamela Dylag, named the bar after Pamela's favorite children's book.

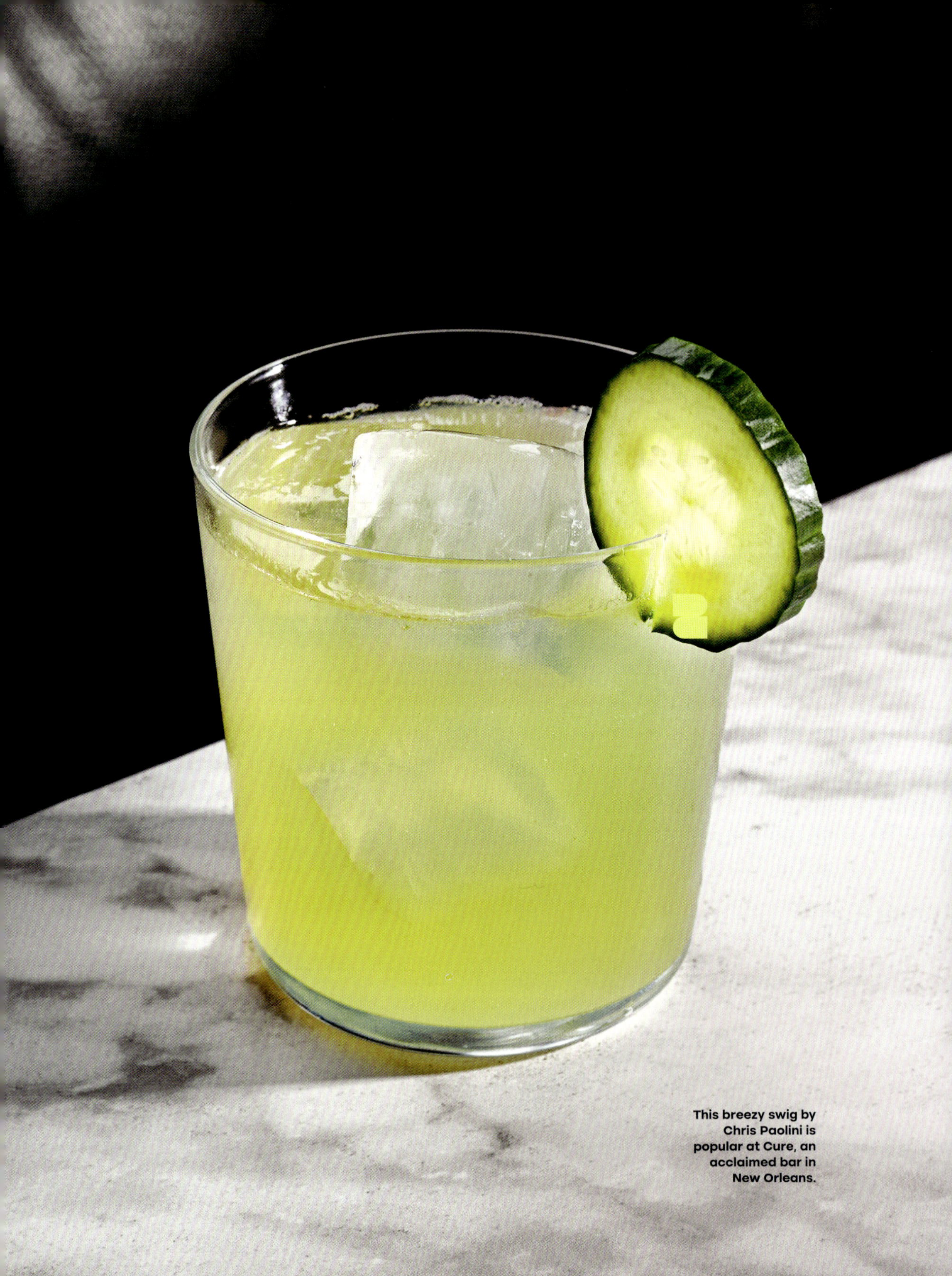

This breezy swig by Chris Paolini is popular at Cure, an acclaimed bar in New Orleans.

Gulfside

Peel from 1 lime (just the outer green part, a.k.a. "lime husk")

Juice of 1 lime

3 slices cucumber

2 sprigs mint

1 oz agave (or to taste)

Ice, for shaking and serving

Soda water, for topping off

7 drops non-alcoholic fruit bitters (such as All the Bitter Orange)

1 cucumber wheel, for serving

1 In shaker, combine lime peel, lime juice, cucumber slices, mint, and agave. Add ice and shake hard for about 10 to 15 seconds, until shaker is frosty.

2 Add fresh ice to a double old-fashioned glass. Strain mocktail over ice. Top with soda water to fill the glass.

3 Top with bitters and garnish with cucumber wheel.

Serves 1. Per serving: 141 cal, 0 g fat, (0 g sat fat), 0 mg chol, 28 mg sodium, 36 g carb, 0 g fiber, 29 g sugar, (28 g added sugar), 0 g pro

INGREDIENT EXPLAINER

Like regular **bitters**, alcohol-free bitters are made with aromatic ingredients like dried orange peel, cardamom, cloves, and coriander. They add depth and complexity to spirit-free spins on old-fashioneds, martinis, and more.

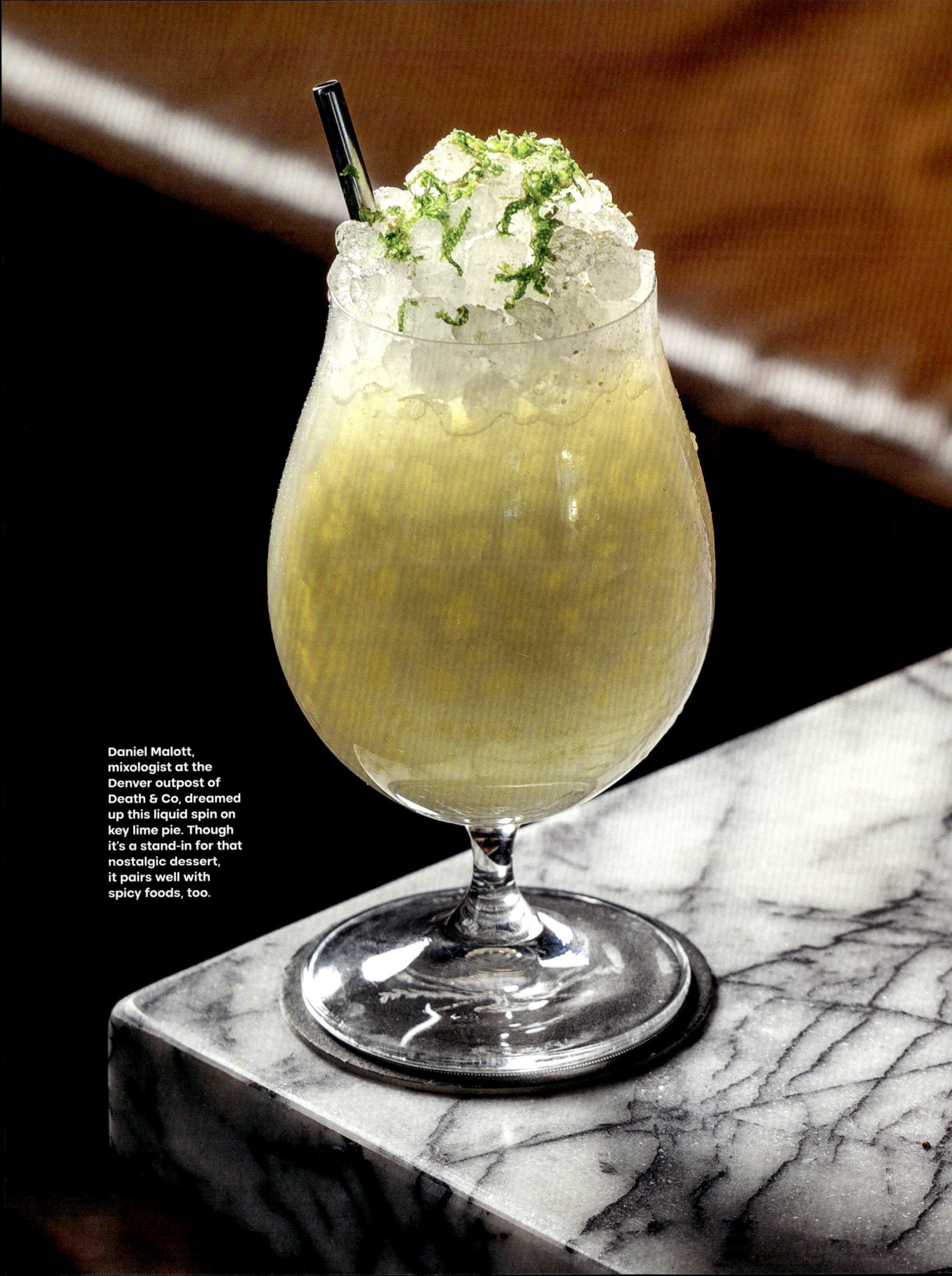

Daniel Malott, mixologist at the Denver outpost of Death & Co, dreamed up this liquid spin on key lime pie. Though it's a stand-in for that nostalgic dessert, it pairs well with spicy foods, too.

FLAVOR PROFILE This is a fun, beachy cocktail with the zest of key lime pie—and totally worth investing in all the special ingredients.

Naysayer

- 1½ oz Seedlip Grove 42 or non-alcoholic gin or tequila
- ½ oz Seedlip Spice 94, or NA gin or tequila
- 1¼ oz calamansi syrup or lime juice
- ¾ oz lime juice
- ¾ oz Greek yogurt
- ½ oz vanilla syrup
- Pebble ice, for shaking and serving
- Grated lime zest, for serving

1 Add all ingredients (except lime zest) to a shaker along with a few pieces of pebble ice and shake briefly, a technique known as whip-shaking. (Pebble ice has a high surface area and works great for chilling without diluting. If you don't have a pebble ice maker, you can crush your own pebble ice with a Lewis ice bag.)

2 Strain drink into a tulip glass. Add a bit of pebble ice and agitate with a swizzle stick to chill the glass. Add another mound of ice and garnish with grated lime zest.

Serves 1. Per serving: 156 cal, 1 g fat, (0.5 g sat fat), 3 mg chol, 19 mg sodium, 35 g carb, 0 g fiber, 32.5 g sugar, (31 g added sugar), 2 g pro

INGREDIENT EXPLAINER

Calamansi syrup is a sweet-and-sour syrup made from the calamansi, a small Asian citrus fruit. You can add a splash to smoothies or drizzle it on pancakes. Find it at Asian grocers or on Amazon.

RAISE THE BAR Seedlip Grove 42 is a citrus-infused NA spirit with notes of blood orange, grapefruit, and lemongrass; **Seedlip Spice 94** is a warm blend of all-spice, cardamom, and citrus.

Char Bear

- 1½ oz non-alcoholic elderflower liqueur (such as Giffard Elderflower)
- ½ oz lemon juice
- ¼ oz agave
- Ice, for shaking and serving
- Club soda, chilled
- Mint sprigs, for serving

1 In shaker with ice, combine all ingredients (except club soda and mint) and shake until frothy.

2 Strain mocktail into rocks glass filled with ice and top with club soda. Garnish with mint sprigs.

Serves 1. Per serving: 87 cal, 0 g fat, (0 g sat fat), 0 mg chol, 26 mg sodium, 21 g carb, 0 g fiber, 19 g sugar, (19 g added sugar), 0 g pro

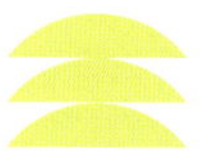

LIFE AFTER ALCOHOL: "I save about $3,500 a year"

Anne was shocked when a friend mentioned she'd gone fully off alcohol. "Over the years we'd had many a chatty dinner over wine, and each of us looked forward to that bracing glass at the end of every workday. Stopping seemed far beyond my reach or even my interest," Anne says. But watching her friend thrive changed that. "She recognized before I did that drinking had become a reflex, an automatic habit, and not a good one." Inspired by her pal's determination, Anne says, "I decided in one unplanned moment at a Sunday brunch to simply stop. Those first few weeks of not drinking were heady. I was excited about my plan." The buddy system helped Anne's switch stick. Another game-changer? Holly Whitaker's *Quit Like a Woman*. "She gave me the phrase 'I don't drink,' which I pressed into service whenever someone offered me a glass. Two years later, Anne is 13 pounds lighter and has zero interest in going back. As a bonus, "I'm saving about $3,500 per year by not buying wine."

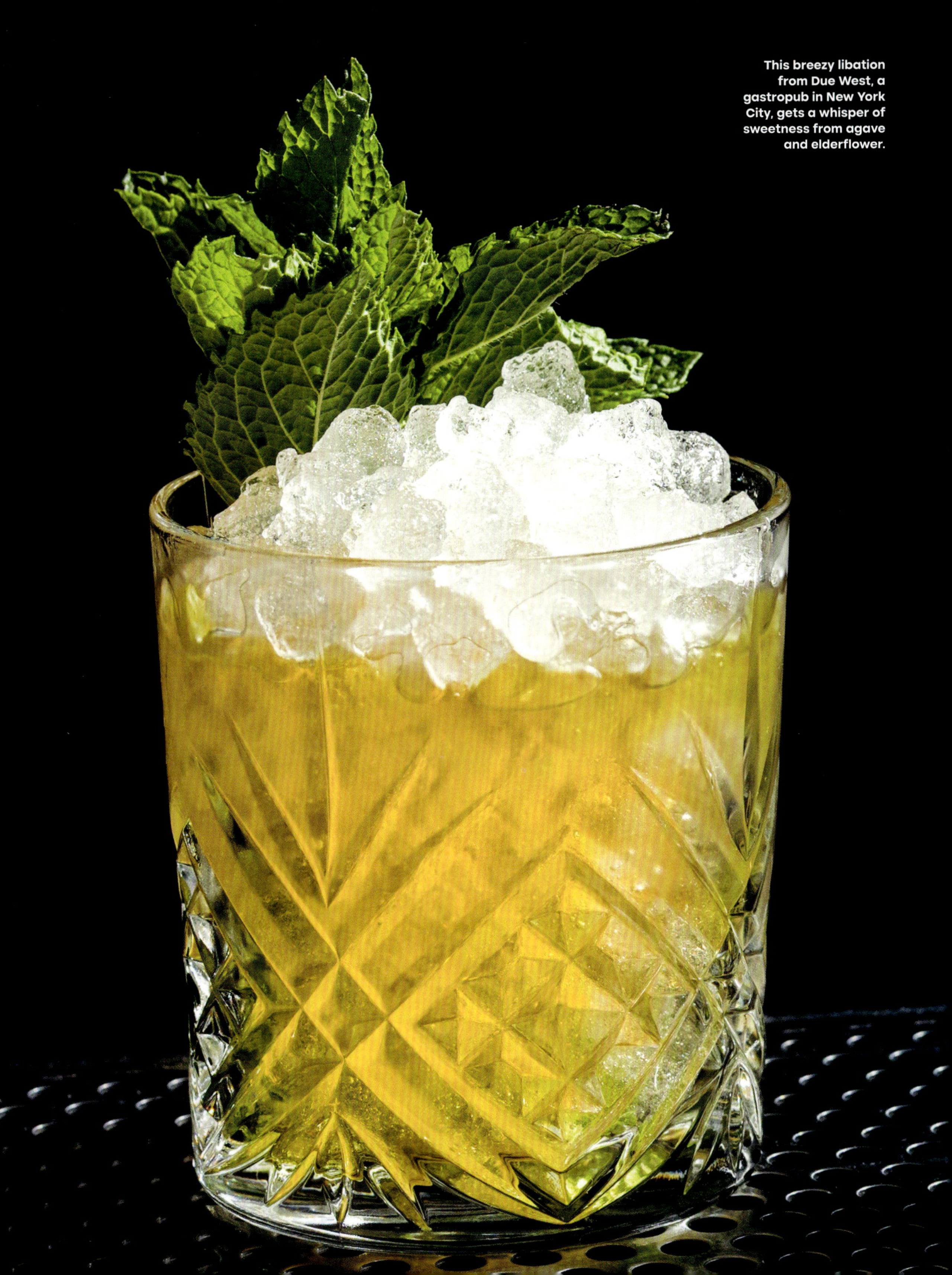

This breezy libation from Due West, a gastropub in New York City, gets a whisper of sweetness from agave and elderflower.

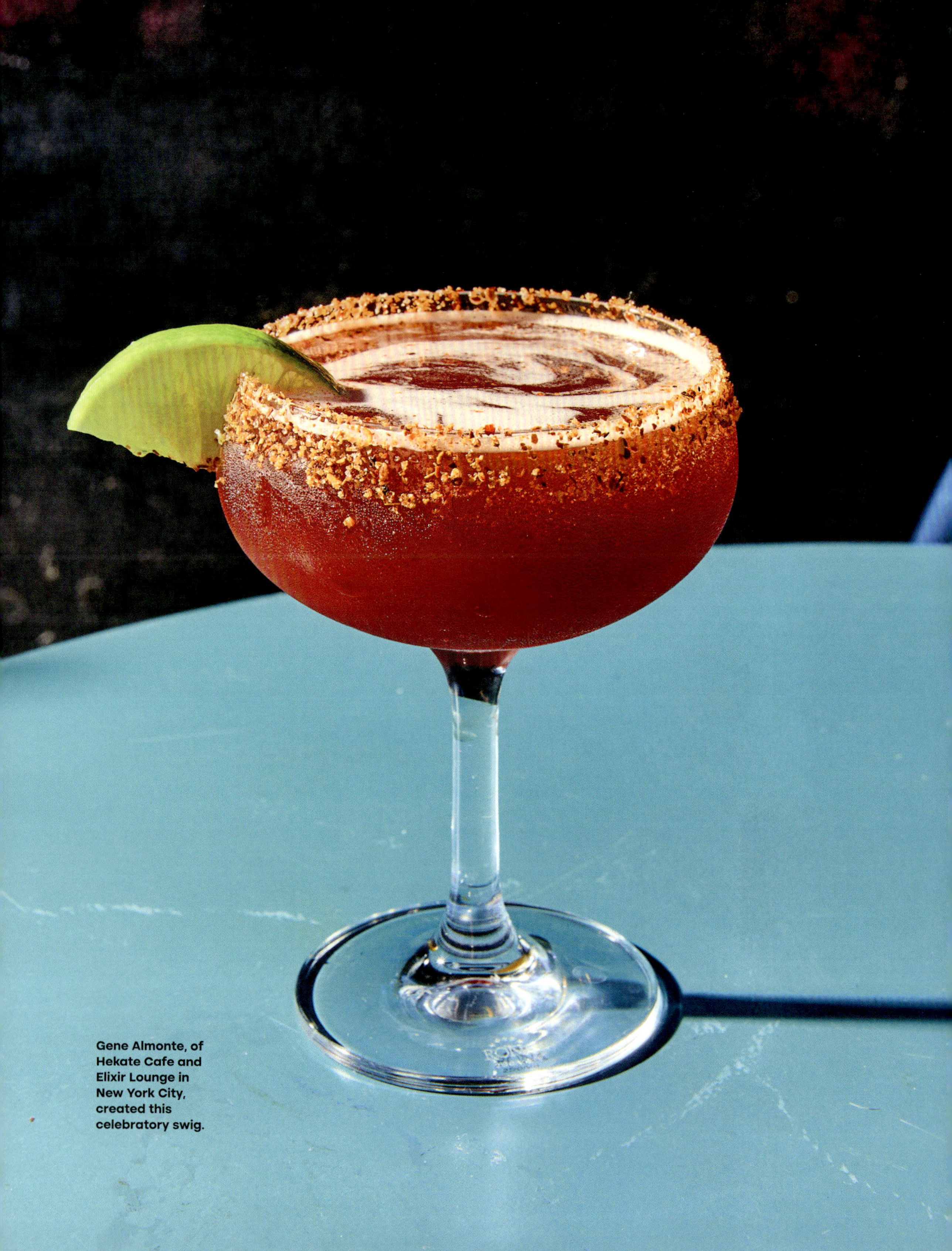

Gene Almonte, of Hekate Cafe and Elixir Lounge in New York City, created this celebratory swig.

FLAVOR PROFILE This sipper brings a bouquet of energetic, juicy notes served with a tart, spicy rim.

Kiss With a Fist

- **2** oz non-alcoholic amaretto liqueur (such as Lyre's Amaretti)
- **2** oz Three Spirit Livener
- **1** oz Ritual Aperitif Alternative
- **½** oz lemon juice
- **½** oz pomegranate juice
- Tajín, for rimming
- Lime slice, for serving

1. In shaker with ice, shake all ingredients (except Tajín and lime slice).

2. Moisten the rim of coupe and dip into a pile of Tajín to coat the rim. Pour drink into glass and garnish with lime slice.

Serves 1. Per serving: About 244 cal, 0 g fat, (0 g sat fat), 0 mg chol, 187 mg sodium, 25 g carb, 0 g fiber, 22 g sugar, (18 g added sugar), 0 g pro

INGREDIENT EXPLAINER

Tajín is a Mexican spice mix of lime, chile peppers, and salt. To rim a glass with it, moisten the rim by running a lime wedge along it, then dip the glass into a plate of Tajín, rotating it to coat it evenly. Tajín is also delicious sprinkled on mango or avocado toast.

RAISE THE BAR Almondy and smooth, **Lyre's Amaretti** warms up spiced wintry mocktails like this. **Three Spirit Livener** delivers flavors of watermelon and ginger, while the **Ritual Aperitif Alternative** tastes of botanicals and bittersweet citrus. Use it to make spirit-free spins on Negronis and other aperitif cocktails.

Positano

- **1** oz Lyre's Italian Spritz or other non-alcoholic Aperol alternative or San Pellegrino Aranciata sparkling beverage
- **6** raspberries, crushed
- **3** basil leaves, cut into ribbons
- **½** oz fresh lemon juice
- Agave to taste (start with ½ oz and add a little at a time until you reach your desired sweetness)
- Ice, for shaking and serving
- Soda water, chilled, for topping off

1 In shaker with ice, combine Lyre's Italian Spritz, raspberries, basil ribbons, lemon juice, and agave. Shake well (at least 30 seconds) and taste; adjust to your desired sweetness, if needed. The ingredients will be blended and raspberries will have burst throughout the drink.

2 Pour into a tall glass. Top with soda water and enjoy.

Serves 1. Per serving: About 163 cal, 0 g fat, (0 g sat fat), 0 mg chol, 3.5 mg sodium, 40 g carb, 1 g fiber, 35 g sugar, (34 g added sugar), 0 g pro

RAISE THE BAR Lyre's Italian Spritz blends the sweetness of orange with the bracing flavor of rhubarb. It's perfect for making a spirit-free Aperol spritz.

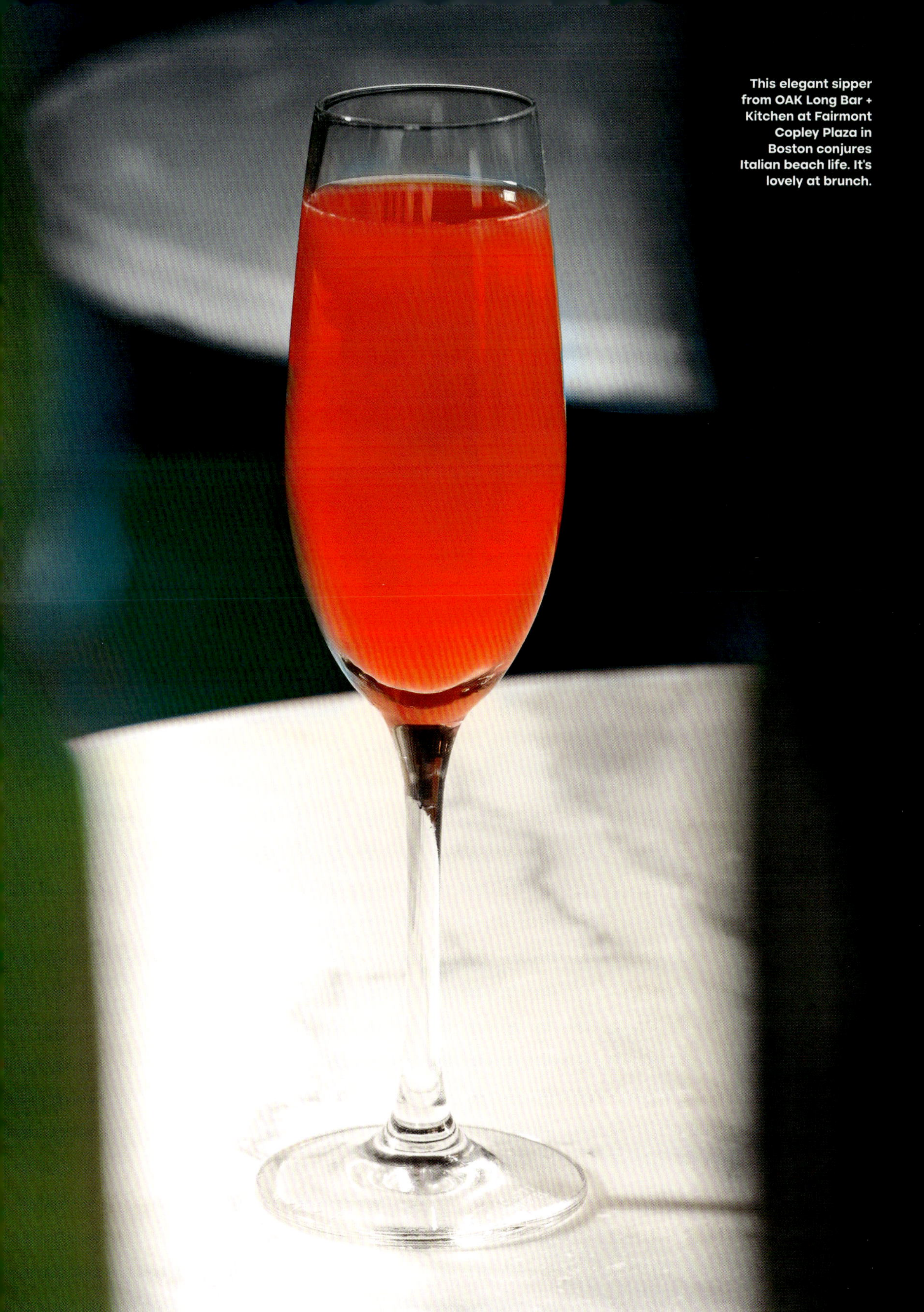

This elegant sipper from OAK Long Bar + Kitchen at Fairmont Copley Plaza in Boston conjures Italian beach life. It's lovely at brunch.

Joe Zino, bar lead at Rootstalk in Breckenridge, Colorado, designed this well-adorned sip.

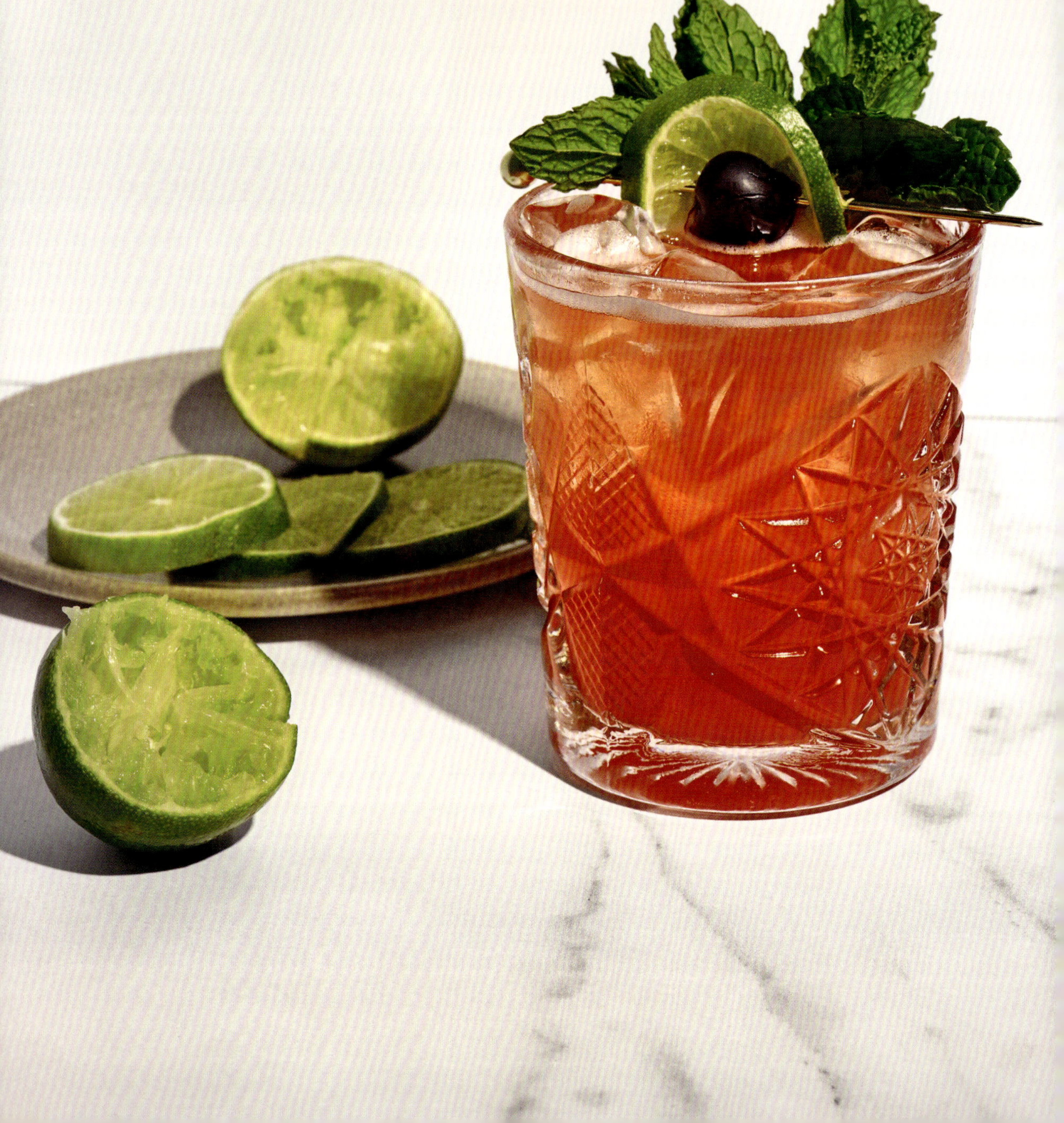

Freebird

- **¼** oz simple syrup (store-bought or use recipe, p. 56)
- **½** oz grenadine (store-bought or use recipe, p. 75)
- **¾** oz lime juice
- **1½** oz pineapple juice
- **1½** oz Giffard Aperitif Bitter
- Ice, for shaking and serving
- **2** oz soda water, chilled
- Pineapple frond (the leaf of a whole pineapple), Luxardo cherry and lime slice on cocktail skewer, and/or mint leaves, for serving, if desired

1. In shaker with ice, shake all ingredients (except soda water and garnishes).
2. Strain into glass filled with ice. Top with soda water.
3. Garnish with pineapple frond, skewered Luxardo cherry and lime slice, or mint, if desired.

Serves 1. Per serving: About 166 cal, 0 g fat, (0 g sat fat), 0 mg chol, 18 mg sodium, 41 g carb, 0 g fiber, 35.5 g sugar, (30.5 g added sugar), 0 g pro

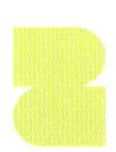

RAISE THE BAR Giffard Aperitif Bitter is a non-alcoholic red syrup that can stand in for bitter red liqueurs like Campari. Add a splash to club soda for a simple, refreshing drink.

Old God Killer

- **2** oz non-alcoholic gin (such as Lyre's)
- **½** oz passionfruit syrup (such as Liquid Alchemist)
- **½** oz cream of coconut
- **¾** oz lemon juice
- Ice, for serving
- Dried orange slice and Luxardo cherry on cocktail skewer, for serving

1 In shaker without ice (known as dry shaking), combine all ingredients and shake for about 10 to 30 seconds.

2 Pour into a rocks glass over ice. Garnish with skewered Luxardo cherry and dried orange slice.

Serves 1. Per serving: About 154 cal, 9 g fat, (8 g sat fat), 0 mg chol, 11 mg sodium, 16 g carb, 2 g fiber, 13 g sugar, (11 g added sugar), 1 g pro

INGREDIENT EXPLAINER

To make **dried orange**, thinly slice an orange ¼ inch thick. Put a cooling tray on a baking sheet, and place the slices on the tray. Bake at 200°F for up to 3 hours. Skewer a slice with a **Luxardo cherry**, a marasca cherry that's been candied using a process without artificial colors and flavors.

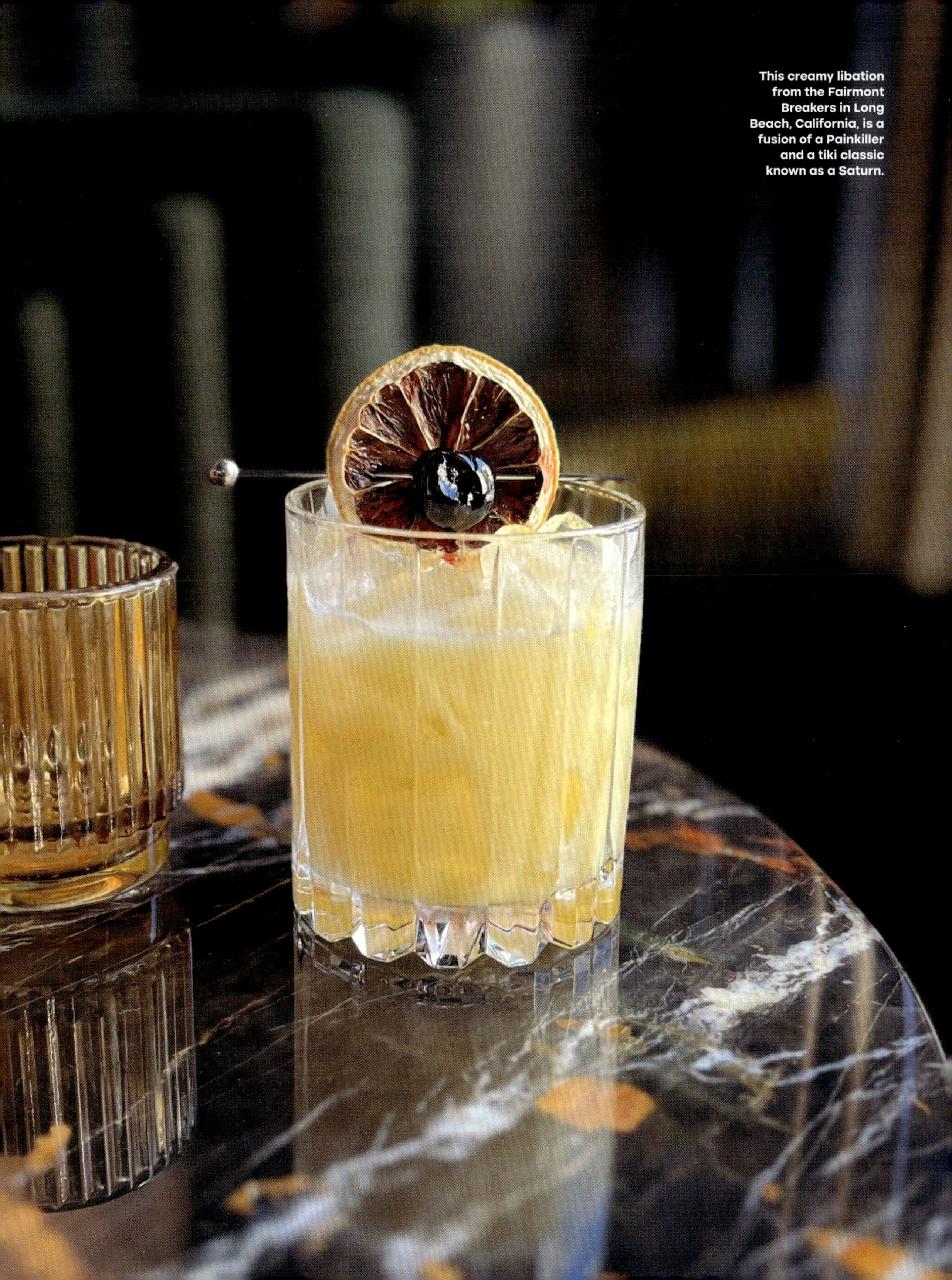

This creamy libation from the Fairmont Breakers in Long Beach, California, is a fusion of a Painkiller and a tiki classic known as a Saturn.

New Twists on Classics

These spirit-free spins rival the originals.

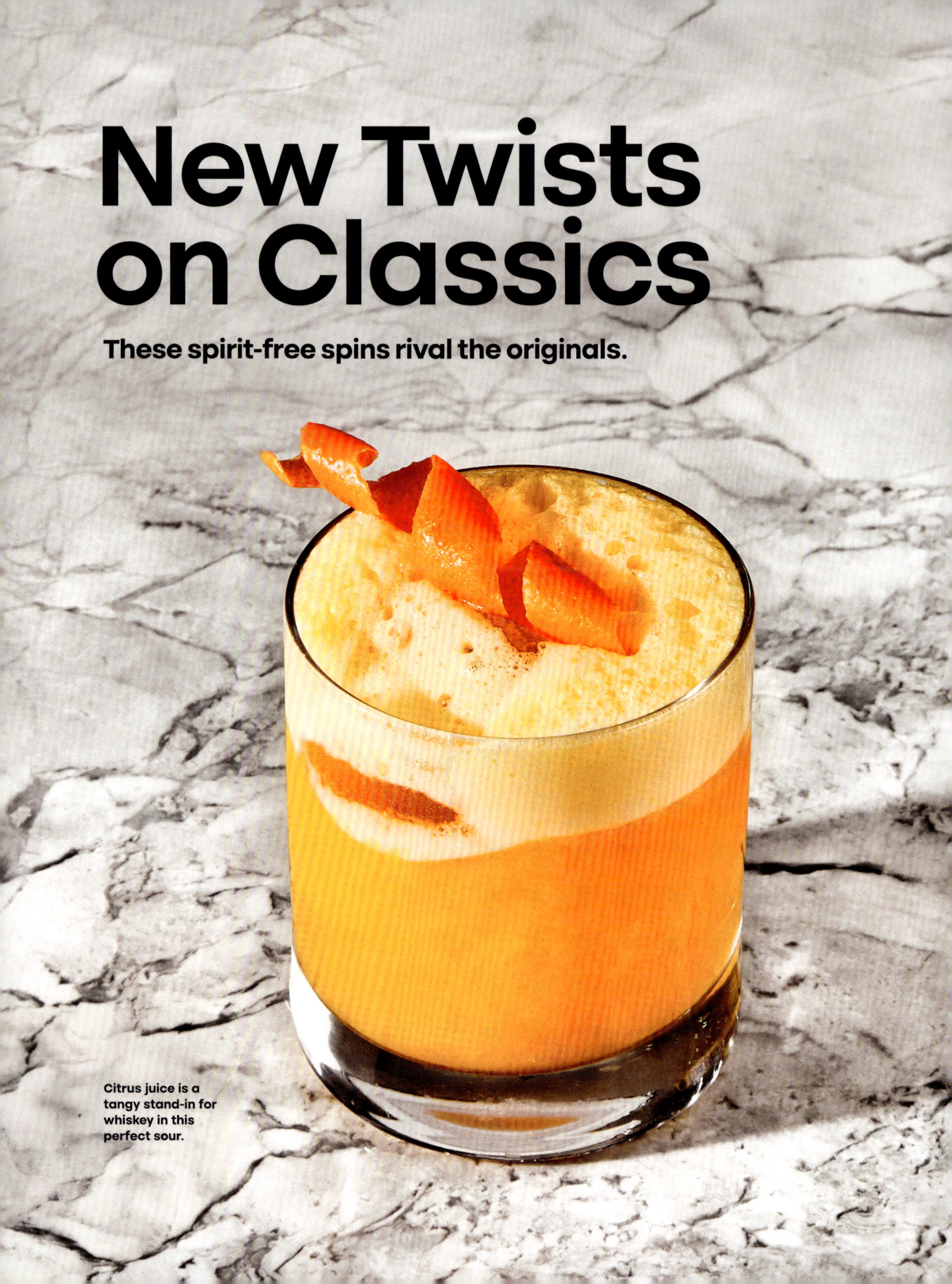

Citrus juice is a tangy stand-in for whiskey in this perfect sour.

FLAVOR PROFILE Zesty citrus and soothing creaminess combine in this spin on the sour.

Tangerine Sour

- **1** cup fresh tangerine or clementine juice (from about 6 tangerines), plus 1 twist tangerine peel, for serving
- **1** Tbsp fresh lemon juice
- **½** tsp pure maple syrup
- **1** Tbsp egg white
- **3** dashes non-alcoholic orange bitters
- Ice, for serving

1. In shaker, combine juices, maple syrup, egg white, and bitters and shake vigorously for 1 minute.

2. Add ice to a rocks glass. Pour over ice and garnish with tangerine twist.

Serves 1. Per serving: About 74 cal, 0.5 g fat (0 g sat), 0 mg chol, 27 mg sodium, 16 g carb, 0.5 g fiber, 15 g sugar (2 g added sugar), 2 g pro

PRO TIP Use a knife or vegetable peeler to cut a 6-inch-long, ½-inch-wide strip of peel from a tangerine (avoid the pith). Wrap the peel around a chopstick or metal straw and hold for 5–10 seconds to set the twist.

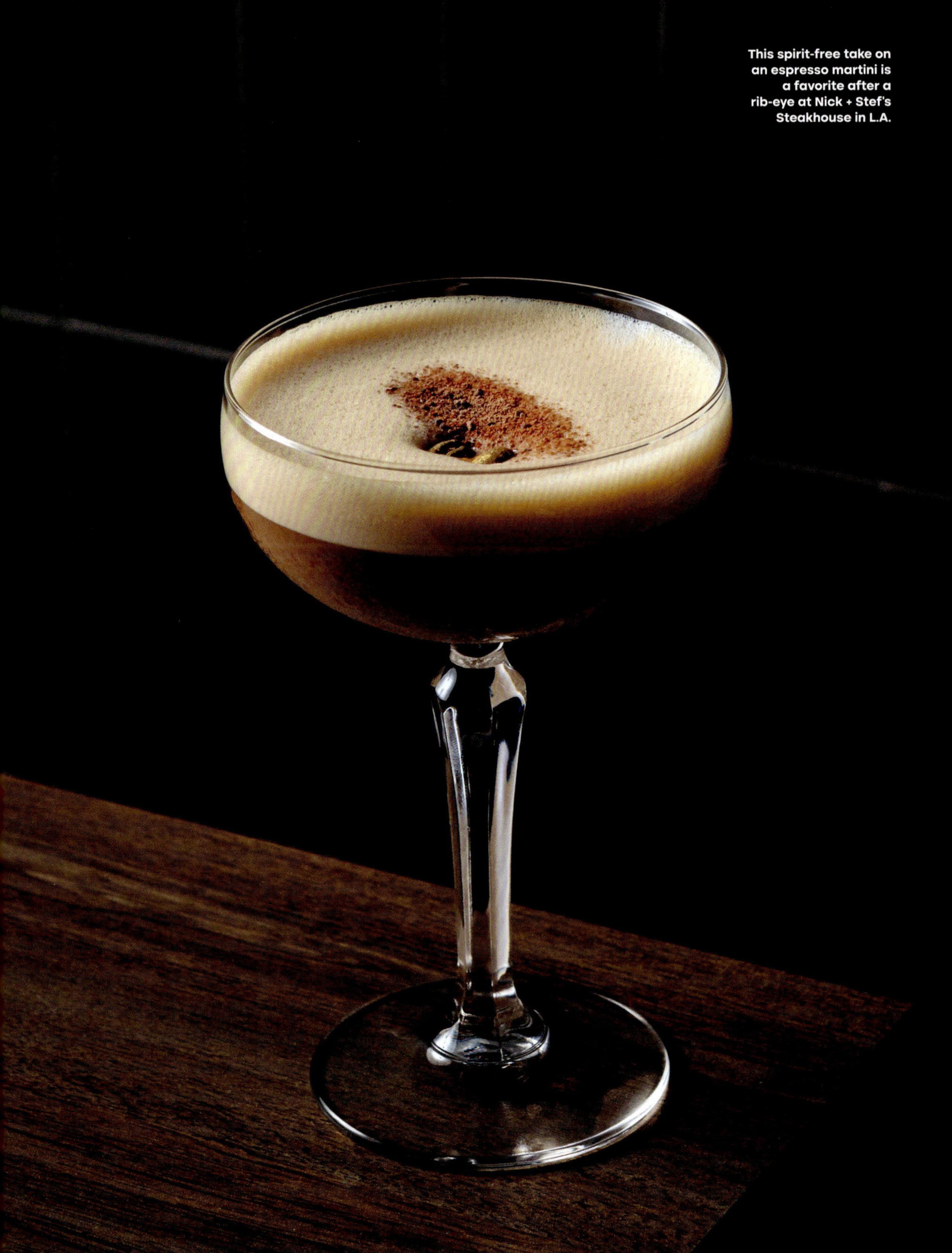

This spirit-free take on an espresso martini is a favorite after a rib-eye at Nick + Stef's Steakhouse in L.A.

Espresso Notini

- **2** oz non-alcoholic tequila (such as Free Spirits)
- **1** oz cold espresso
- **½** oz agave

1. In shaker with ice, combine all ingredients and shake until the shaker is frosty.
2. Double strain into martini glass or coupe.

Serves 1. Per serving: About 69 cal, 0 g fat, (0 g sat fat), 0 mg chol, 21 mg sodium, 18 g carb, 0 g fiber, 17 g sugar, (17 g added sugar), 0 g pro

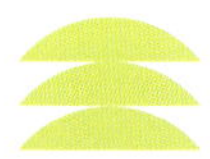

LIFE AFTER ALCOHOL: "I found freedom"

"From my first sip at 14, I knew I liked alcohol more than others," Lori recalls. Her partying 20s gave way to wine nights in her 30s. "Alcohol made everything—dark nights, sunny days, celebrations—seem better," she says. By her late 30s, something shifted when she discovered Marc Maron's podcast. "He made sobriety aspirational—like an enlightened state. Not the white-knuckled punishment, I'd imagined." She also began dating someone who didn't drink. "It was the relationship I'd always wanted, until it wasn't. I'd considered before that drinking could be keeping me from love. Since my teens, I'd used alcohol to regulate my emotions. How could I be intimate with someone when I'd spent over two decades disconnecting from myself? Suddenly, I saw that alcohol wasn't bringing me happiness—it was what kept me in the dark." Lori knew she didn't want to drink anymore. She returned to therapy and practiced being present, even in discomfort. "I'd worried about feeling loss, and I did—of a weight I hadn't known I was carrying. Without the noise of alcohol, I could finally listen to myself."

Guava Margarita

- Lime wedges, for rimming and serving
- Salt, for rimming, if desired
- Ice, for shaking and serving
- ½ cup guava nectar
- 3 Tbsp fresh orange juice
- 2 Tbsp fresh lime juice
- Lime slice, for serving

1. Rub rim of a glass with lime slice then dip in salt to coat, if desired. Add ice to glass.
2. Fill shaker with ice, add juices, and shake until shaker is frosty.
3. Strain into salt-rimmed glass. Garnish with lime slice.

Serves 1. Per serving: About 78 cal, 0 g fat (0 g sat), 0 mg chol, 486 mg sodium, 20 g carb, 1 g fiber, 14.5 g sugar (0 g added sugar), 1 g pro

Make a Pitcher

(SERVES 6–8)

COMBINE 1½ cups guava nectar, 9 Tbsp (just over ½ cup) fresh orange juice, and 6 Tbsp (about ⅓ cup + 1 Tbsp) fresh lime juice in large shaker. **ADD** a big scoop of ice and shake or stir well to combine and chill. **TO SERVE** Fill salt-rimmed glasses with fresh ice and add mocktail. Garnish each glass with lime wedge.

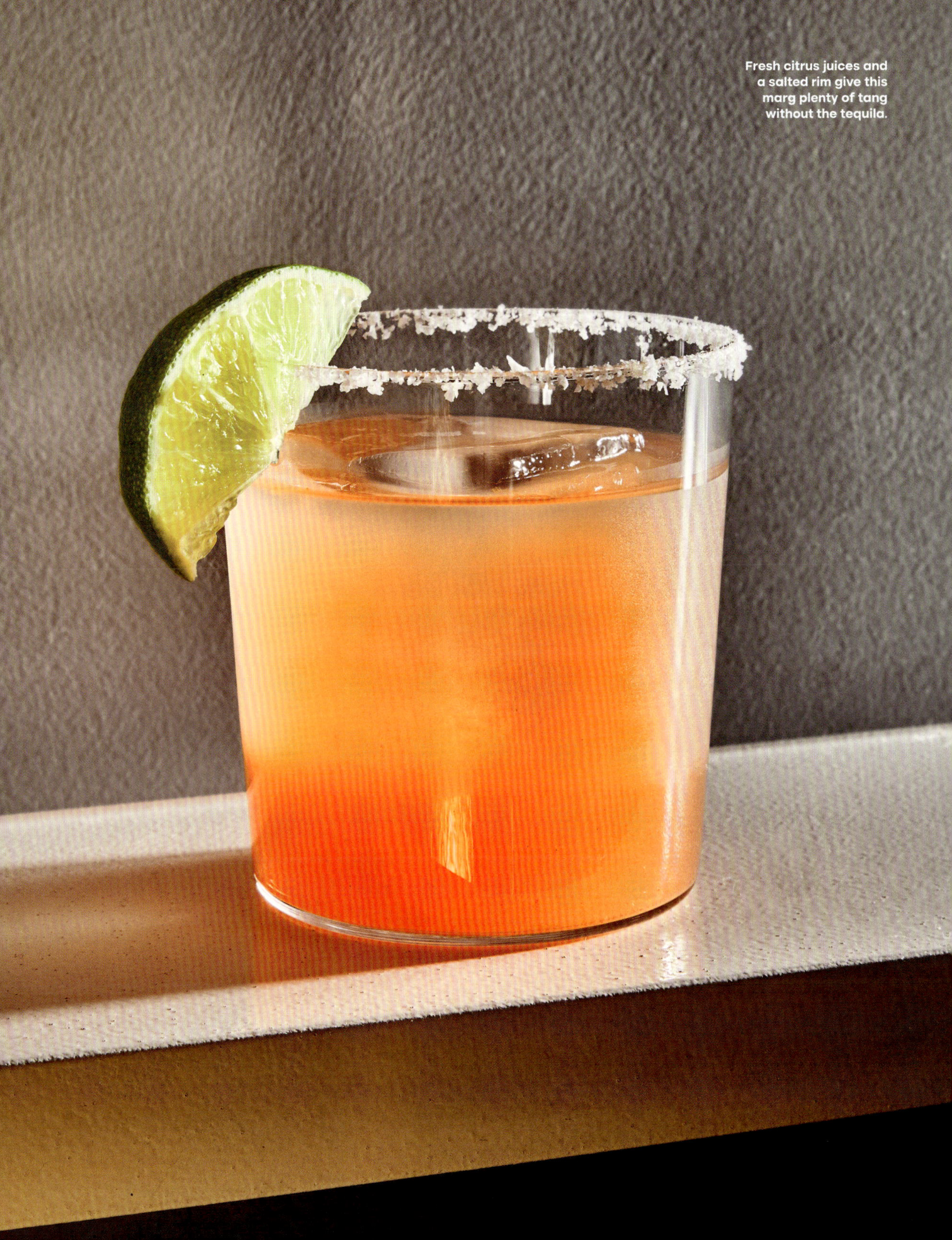

Fresh citrus juices and a salted rim give this marg plenty of tang without the tequila.

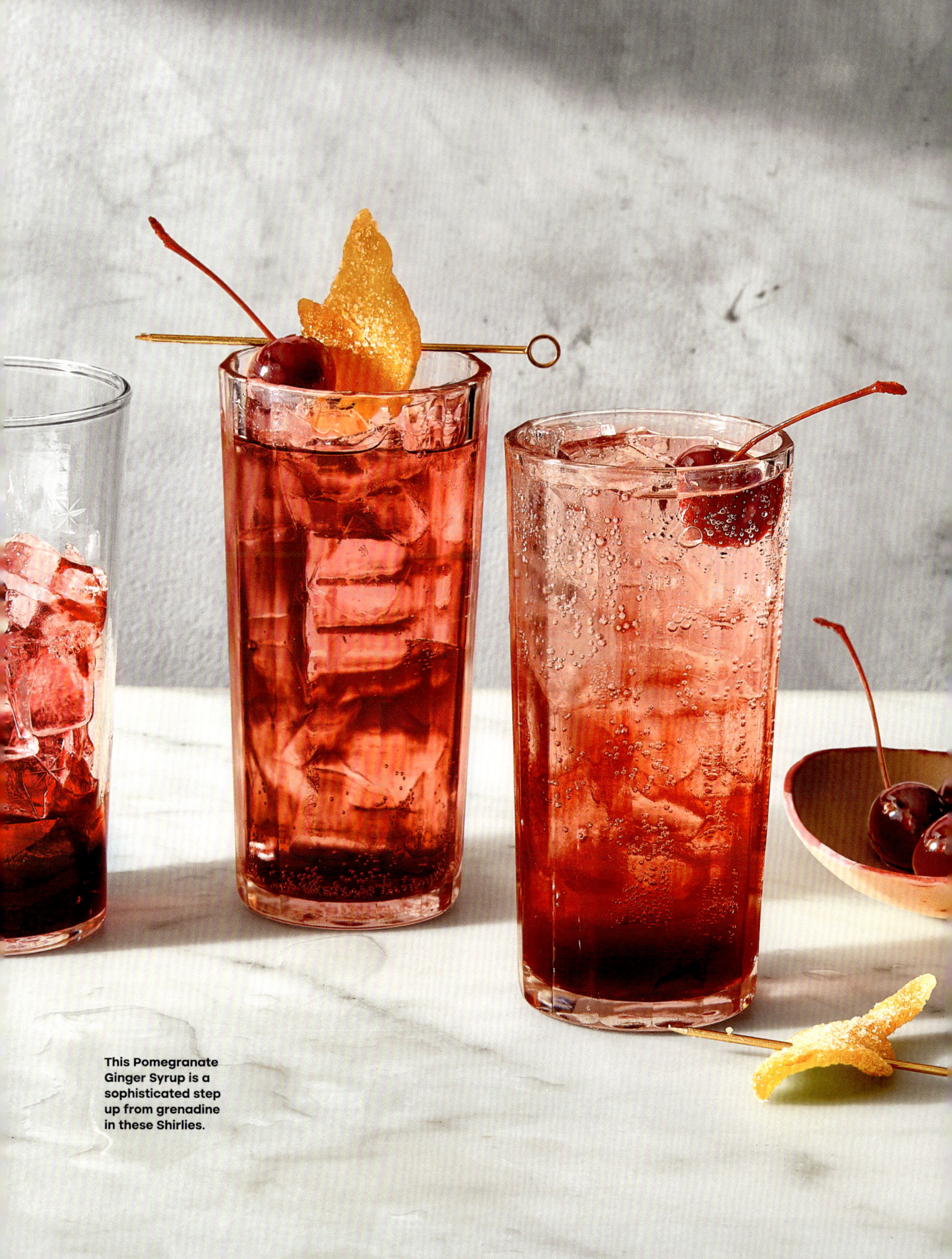

This Pomegranate Ginger Syrup is a sophisticated step up from grenadine in these Shirlies.

Gingery Shirley Temple

1 Tbsp Pomegranate Ginger Syrup (recipe below)

Ice, for serving

Club soda, chilled, for topping off

Luxardo cherry and candied ginger, for serving

Fill a Collins glass with ice. Add Pomegranate Ginger Syrup, top with club soda, and stir. Garnish with Luxardo cherry and candied ginger.

Serves 1. Per serving: About 44 cal, 0 g fat, (0 g sat fat), 0 mg chol, 50.5 mg sodium, 11 g carb, 0 g fiber, 11 g sugar, (9 g added sugar), 0 g pro

Pomegranate Ginger Syrup

COMBINE 3/4 cup sugar, 3/4 cup pomegranate juice, and 1/2-inch piece fresh ginger, thinly sliced, in small saucepan. **HEAT**, stirring once halfway through, until sugar dissolves, about 12 minutes. **REMOVE** from heat and let cool to room temperature, about 15 minutes; strain into jar. Makes 1 cup.

Virgin Pineapple Mule

- ¼ cup pineapple juice
- 1 Tbsp lime juice, plus lime or lemon wedge for serving
- 1 tsp balsamic vinegar
- ¼ cup ginger beer, chilled
- Ice, for serving
- Mint sprig and blackberries on cocktail skewer, for serving

1. In liquid measuring cup, stir pineapple juice, lime juice, and balsamic vinegar until uniform in color.

2. Pour into tall ice-filled glass; gently stir in ginger beer. Garnish with lime or lemon wedge, mint sprig, and blackberries, if desired.

Serves 1. Per serving: About 67 cal, 0 g fat (0 g sat), 0 mg chol, 9 mg sodium, 17 g carb, 0 g fiber, 13.5 g sugar (6 g added sugar), 0 g pro

Make a Pitcher

(SERVES 6–8)

STIR together 1½ cups pineapple juice, 6 Tbsp fresh lime juice (about 3 limes), and 2 Tbsp balsamic vinegar in large pitcher or mixing bowl until fully combined. **CHILL** mixture in fridge until ready to serve. Just before serving, stir in 1½ to 2 cups chilled ginger beer. **FILL** tall glasses with ice and add mixture. Garnish each glass with mint sprig, lime or lemon wedge, and skewer of blackberries.

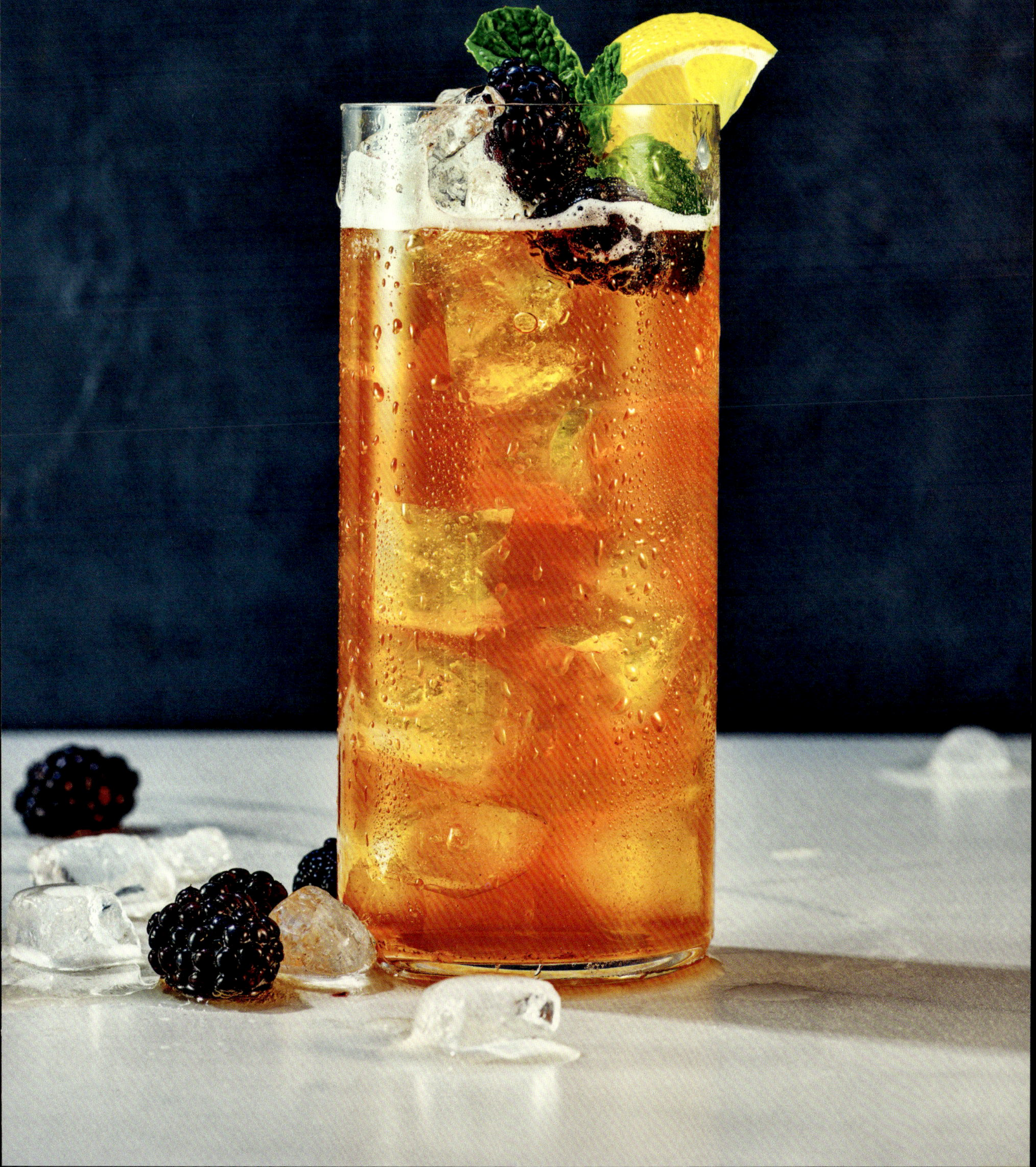

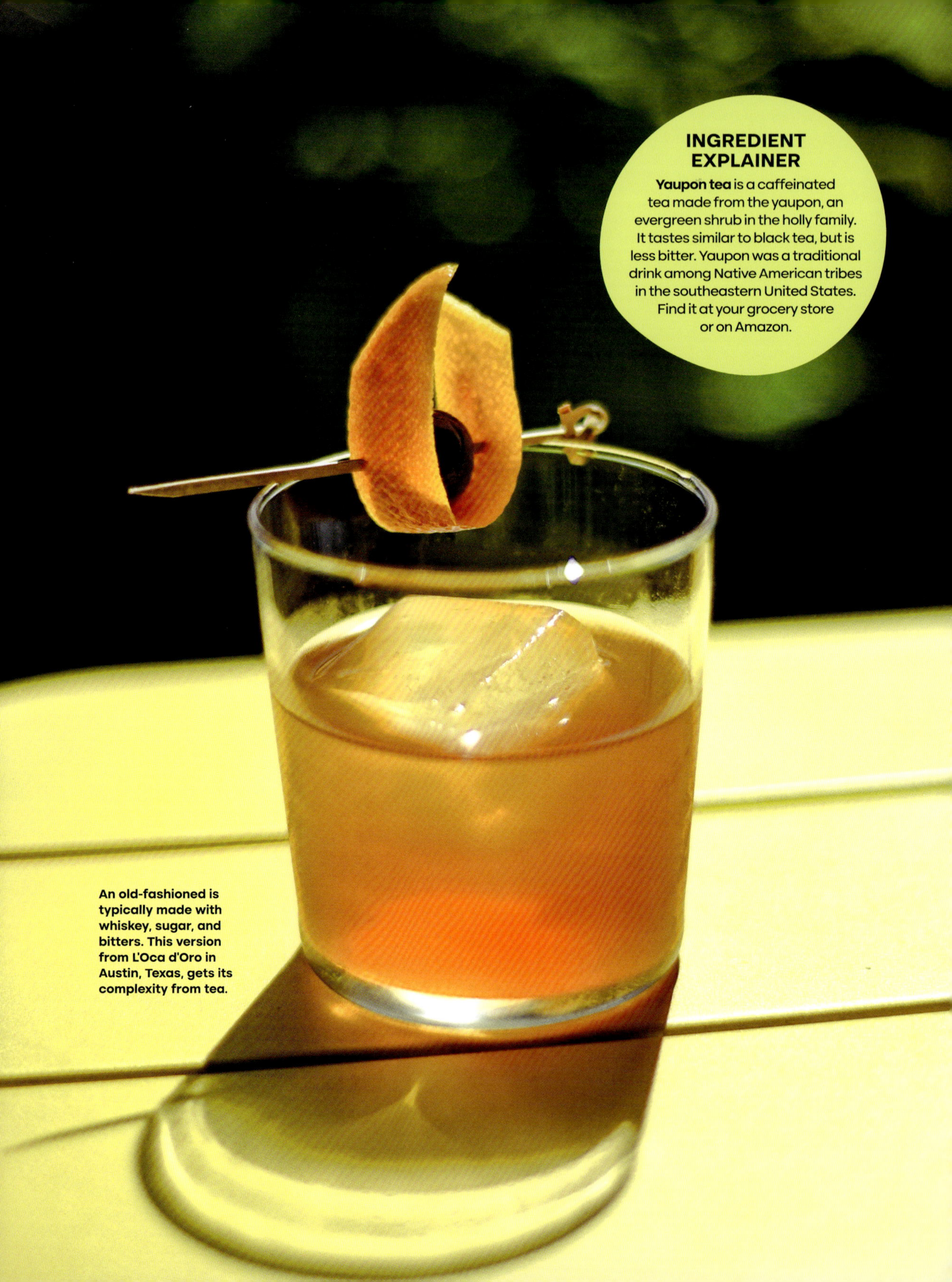

INGREDIENT EXPLAINER

Yaupon tea is a caffeinated tea made from the yaupon, an evergreen shrub in the holly family. It tastes similar to black tea, but is less bitter. Yaupon was a traditional drink among Native American tribes in the southeastern United States. Find it at your grocery store or on Amazon.

An old-fashioned is typically made with whiskey, sugar, and bitters. This version from L'Oca d'Oro in Austin, Texas, gets its complexity from tea.

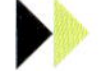

FLAVOR PROFILE Herby and warm-toned tea and a duo of bitters give this bev bite.

Dry County Old-Fashioned

- **1¼** tsp Orange-Yaupon Cordial (recipe below)
- **4** dashes non-alcoholic aromatic bitters
- **4** dashes NA orange bitters (such as All the Bitter brand)
- **3** oz cold yaupon tea in dark roast (brewed per package directions)
- Large ice cube, for serving
- Orange peel and Luxardo cherry on cocktail skewer, for serving

1. Add Orange-Yaupon Cordial to the bottom of rocks glass along with bitters. Top with the tea and a large ice cube. Stir with a bar spoon, about 30 turns.

2. Garnish with skewered orange peel and Luxardo cherry.

Serves 1. Per serving: About 56 cal, 0 g fat, (0 g sat fat), 0 mg chol, 1 mg sodium, 14 g carb, 0 g fiber, 12 g sugar, (12 g added sugar), 0 g pro

Orange-Yaupon Cordial

COMBINE 2 cups brewed yaupon tea (or black tea), ¾ cup orange juice, ¼ cup lemon juice, and 3½ cups sugar in small saucepan. Add half of a whole orange. **COOK** on medium high heat until mixture begins to bubble. Stir; simmer for 3 or 4 minutes. **REMOVE** from heat, remove and discard orange, add 6 or 7 mint leaves, and cover saucepan with towel. Allow to steep for 10 to 15 minutes. **STRAIN** cordial into jar and chill.

Scott Ruggiero, a mixologist at Death & Co in Denver, created this take on the Negroni, which pairs floral, bitter elements with espresso.

LOW-SUGAR SIPPER!

Wheeling & Dealing

- 1½ oz non-alcoholic gin (such as Lyre's)
- 1 oz NA red wine
- ½ oz NA red vermouth (such as Martini & Rossi Vibrante)
- 1 tsp espresso (brewed and cooled) or cold brew concentrate
- Ice, for shaking
- Large ice cube, for serving
- Grapefruit slice, for serving

1. In shaker with ice, combine all ingredients (except grapefruit slice) and shake until shaker is frosty.

2. Pour into old-fashioned glass with large ice cube. Garnish with grapefruit slice.

Serves 1. Per serving: About 27.5 cal, 0 g fat, (0 g sat fat), 0 mg chol, 5 mg sodium, 7 g carb, 0 g fiber, 4.5 g sugar, (4.5 g added sugar), 0 g pro

RAISE THE BAR Non-alcoholic red vermouth, such as **Martini & Rossi Vibrante**, brings bittersweet complexity to faux Negronis. It's also lovely just paired with tonic water.

FLAVOR PROFILE This dreamy sangria is made with the warm notes of non-alcoholic spirits and red wine.

Sleepy Sangria

- **1** oz Three Spirit Nightcap
- **1** oz Sparkplug Syrup (recipe below)
- **2** oz non-alcoholic dark rum (such as Caleño Dark and Spicy)
- **½** oz lemon juice
- **½** oz lime juice
- **¼** oz sparkling water
- Ice, for serving
- NA red wine, for topping off
- Apple slice and orange slice, for serving

1 Build all ingredient in wineglass filled with ice, in the order given. Don't stir. Top with red wine.

2 Garnish with an apple slice and orange slice.

Serves 1. Per serving: About 102 cal, 0 g fat, (0 g sat fat), 0 mg chol, 28 mg sodium, 27 g carb, 0 g fiber, 24 g sugar, (23 g added sugar), 0 g pro

RAISE THE BAR Three Spirit Nightcap is a woodsy blend of valerian root, hops, and lemon balm, with notes of maple, vanilla, and spice. It's also pleasant served neat or over ice with a splash of sparkling water.

Sparkplug Syrup

BRING 2 cups water to boil. **ADD** 2 cups sugar and stir until dissolved. **ADD** a small handful of chopped fresh ginger and 10 to 15 cinnamon sticks. **SIMMER** on low heat for 30 minutes. **STRAIN** into a container and allow to cool before using.

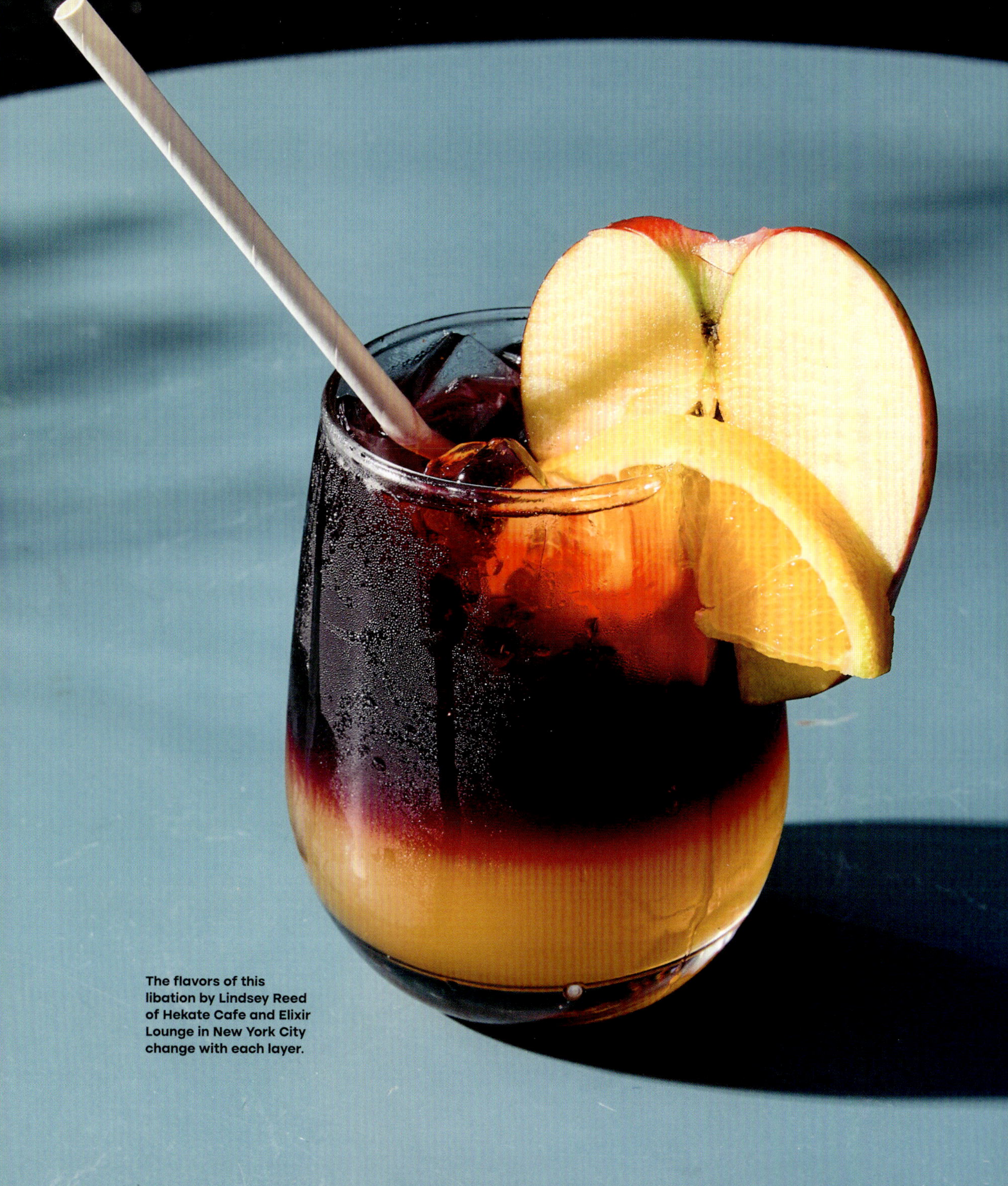

The flavors of this libation by Lindsey Reed of Hekate Cafe and Elixir Lounge in New York City change with each layer.

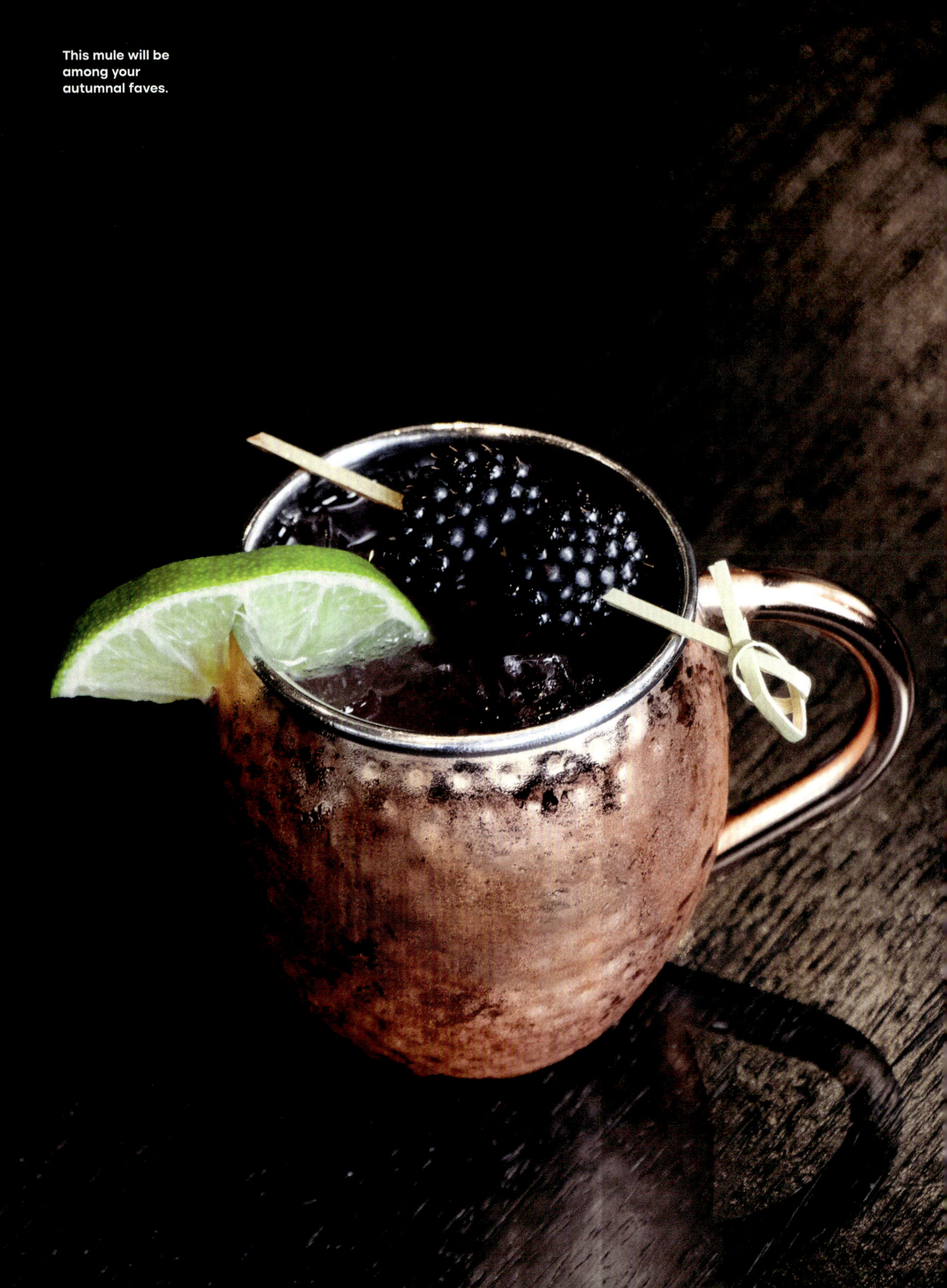

This mule will be among your autumnal faves.

Blackberry Mule

- ¼ oz Blackberry Puree (recipe below)
- ½ oz lime juice
- Ice, for serving
- Ginger beer, chilled, for topping off
- Blackberries on cocktail skewer and lime slice, for serving

In copper mug, add Blackberry Puree and lime juice. Add ice and top with ginger beer. Garnish with skewered blackberries and lime slice.

Serves 1. Per serving: About 101 cal, 0 g fat, (0 g sat fat), 0 mg chol, 0.5 mg sodium, 26 g carb, 0 g fiber, 25 g sugar, (24 g added sugar), 0 g pro

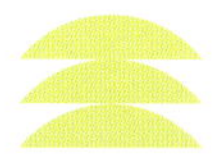

LIFE AFTER ALCOHOL: "I couldn't be happier"

Kate looked like she had it all together. But behind closed doors, there was a pattern she couldn't ignore. "I wasn't pouring vodka on my cornflakes or drinking and driving. But every night, I had this irresistible urge to hit the self-destruct button," she says. After a particularly brutal hangover, she realized she had six months until she turned 30. "Taking my problem drinking with me into the next decade seemed incredibly sad," she says. "I read books, listened to podcasts, and educated myself about alcohol and addiction. I reached out to others who were sober and—shockingly—enjoying life. I'm five years sober now, and I couldn't be happier. Sobriety is about creating a life that's so good, you don't need to numb out from it."

Blackberry Puree

PUREE 2 pints blackberries in food processor until smooth. **ADD** 1 Tbsp sugar and puree again. **STRAIN** puree through a fine-mesh sieve. Use immediately or refrigerate.

Savory Sips

Spice, salt, and some heat up ahead!

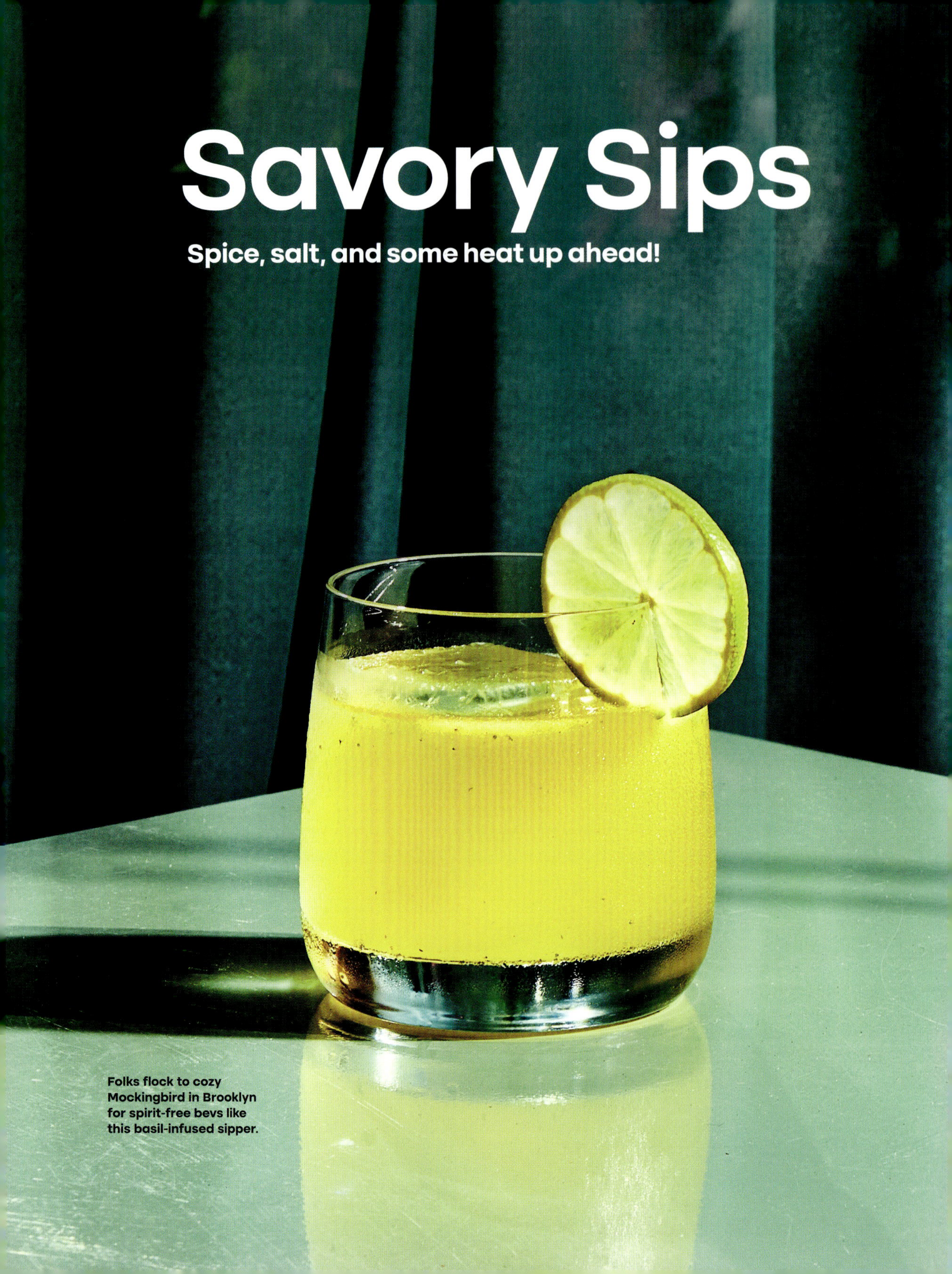

Folks flock to cozy Mockingbird in Brooklyn for spirit-free bevs like this basil-infused sipper.

FLAVOR PROFILE The herby, citrusy mocktail gets smoke from the mezcal and heat from the pepper.

Smoke Show

- **1** serrano pepper, cut into ¼-inch slices and deseeded
- **4–5** cilantro leaves
- **2** oz non-alcoholic mezcal, preferably spicy (such as Abstinence Cape Agave)
- **¾** oz lime juice
- **¾** oz orange juice
- **1** oz Basil Syrup (recipe below)
- **2–3** dashes NA orange bitters or additional ¼ oz orange juice
- Ice, for shaking and serving
- Lime wheel, for serving

1 In shaker, muddle serrano pepper with cilantro. Add remaining ingredients (except lime wheel) and shake with ice until shaker is frosty.

2 Add fresh ice to a rocks glass. Strain mocktail over ice. Garnish with a lime wheel.

Serves 1. Per serving: About 96 cal, 0 g fat, (0 g sat fat), 0 mg chol, 8 mg sodium, 24 g carb, 0 g fiber, 20 g sugar, (18 g added sugar), 0 g pro

Basil Syrup

COMBINE 1 cup water, 1 cup white cane sugar, and 1 cup torn basil leaves in small saucepan. **BRING** to a boil, then reduce to a simmer, 1 minute, until sugar is dissolved. **REMOVE** from heat and let steep for 20 minutes. **STRAIN** syrup into glass jar and store in the fridge for up to 2 weeks.

FLAVOR PROFILE This sip is spicy with a hint of pepper and smokiness.

Firepit Nights

- **2½** oz non-alcoholic whiskey (such as Monday)
- **1** oz lime juice
- **1** oz Rosemary Syrup (recipe below)
- **½** oz juiced bell pepper and habanero (3 of each pepper blended with 1 cup water) or at least 3 dashes NA spicy bitters, (like Fee Brothers)
- Ice, for shaking and serving
- Sparkling water, chilled, for topping off
- Scorched rosemary sprig, for serving, if desired

1 In shaker with ice, add all ingredients (except sparkling water and rosemary sprig) and shake until shaker is frosty.

2 Add fresh ice to a tall glass. Strain mocktail over ice.

3 Top with sparkling water to temper spiciness. Garnish with scorched rosemary sprig, if desired. (Let the rosemary dry a day or two, so it's easy to scorch with a lighter. Do this over the sink and quickly blow out the flame.)

Serves 1. Per serving: About 87 cal, 0 g fat, (0 g sat fat), 0 mg chol, 14 mg sodium, 23 g carb, 0 g fiber, 19 g sugar, (18.5 g added sugar), 0 g pro

Rosemary Syrup

STEEP a few sprigs of rosemary in 1 cup hot water until they turn reddish green (preferably on a low simmer on the stove). **MIX** in 1 cup agave or 1 cup sugar. Let mixture cool. **STRAIN** through fine-mesh sieve into a container or jar. **STORE** in the fridge for up to 1 week.

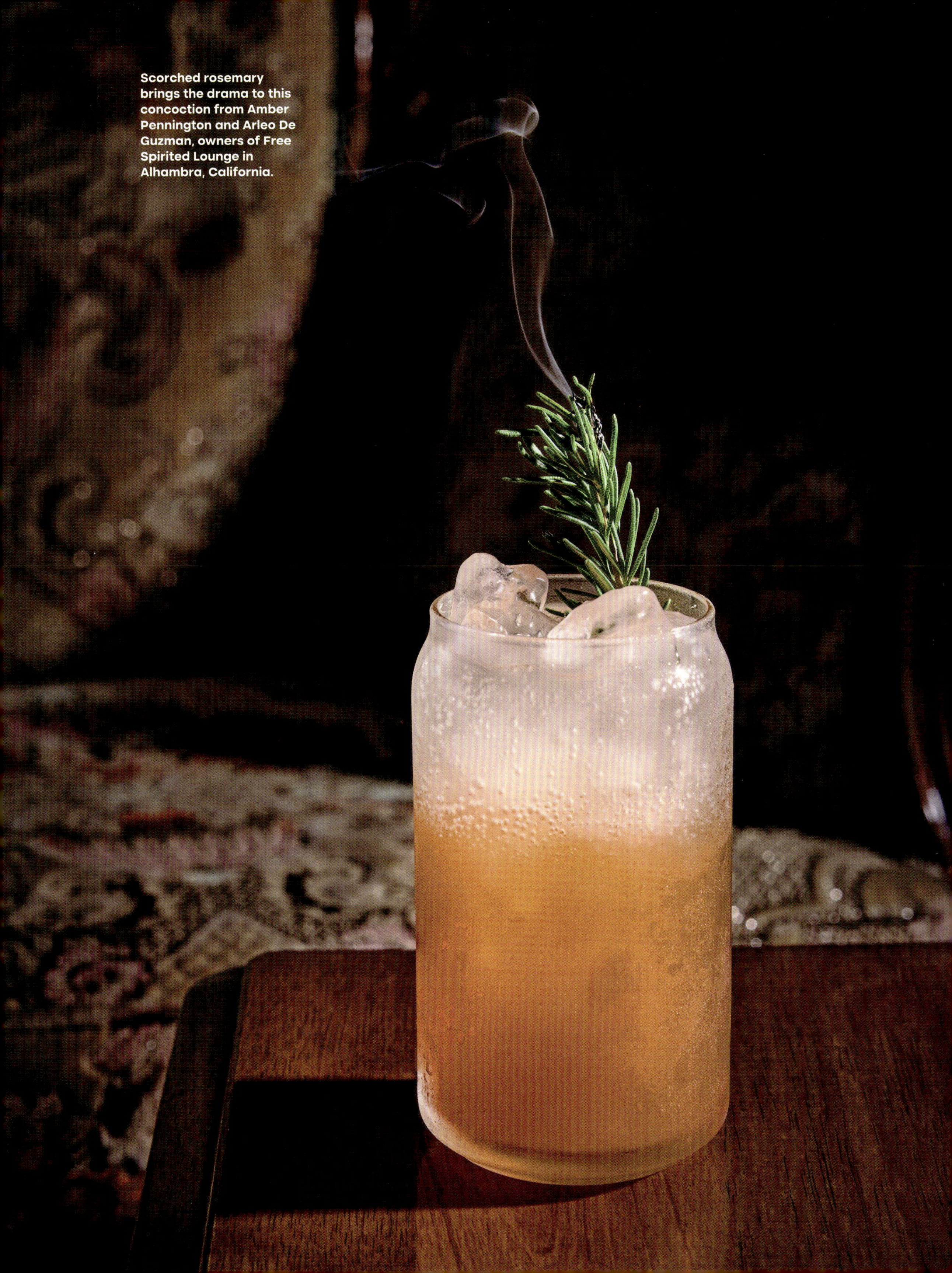

Scorched rosemary brings the drama to this concoction from Amber Pennington and Arleo De Guzman, owners of Free Spirited Lounge in Alhambra, California.

FLAVOR PROFILE Honey syrup gives this frothy sip a whisper of sweetness.

Unknown Legend

- **2** oz grapefruit juice
- **1** oz lime juice
- **2** oz aquafaba (starchy liquid in a can of chickpeas)
- **2** oz Burnt Honey Bay Leaf Syrup (recipe below)
- Ice, for shaking
- Large ice, for serving
- Smoked paprika, for serving

1 In shaker, add all ingredients (except ice and paprika) and shake hard for about 15 to 30 seconds. Add ice to shaker and shake again until shaker is frosty.

2 Strain mocktail into a chilled rocks glass with 1 big rock in it (you can purchase a rock ice mold). If you don't have rock ice, pour mocktail into a stemmed glass like a Nick and Nora or a coupe straight up. Sprinkle with smoked paprika.

Serves 1. Per serving: About 191 cal, 0 g fat, (0 g sat fat), 0 mg chol, 6 mg sodium, 50 g carb, 0 g fiber, 46 g sugar, (40 g added sugar), 1 g pro

Burnt Honey Bay Leaf Syrup

HEAT 1 Tbsp water, 1 cup honey, and 3 bay leaves over medium heat in medium saucepan until it starts to bubble. (You want the honey to change to a darker shade to get that lightly burnt caramel flavor.) Remove from heat. **ADD** ¾ cup water immediately to the honey. It will bubble up a lot so add it carefully. **REMOVE** bay leaves. **POUR** syrup into a glass jar and keep in the fridge for up to a month.

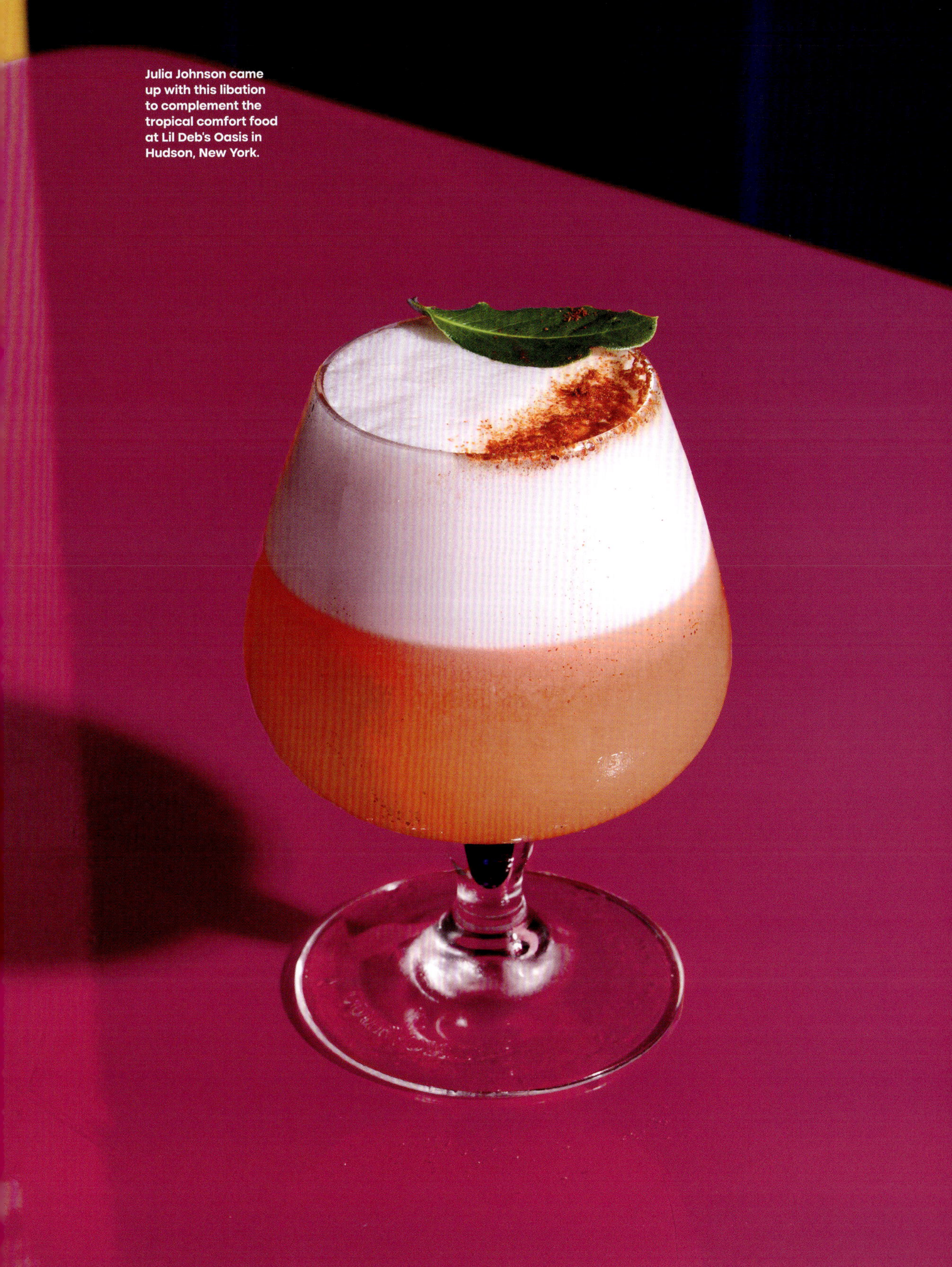

Julia Johnson came up with this libation to complement the tropical comfort food at Lil Deb's Oasis in Hudson, New York.

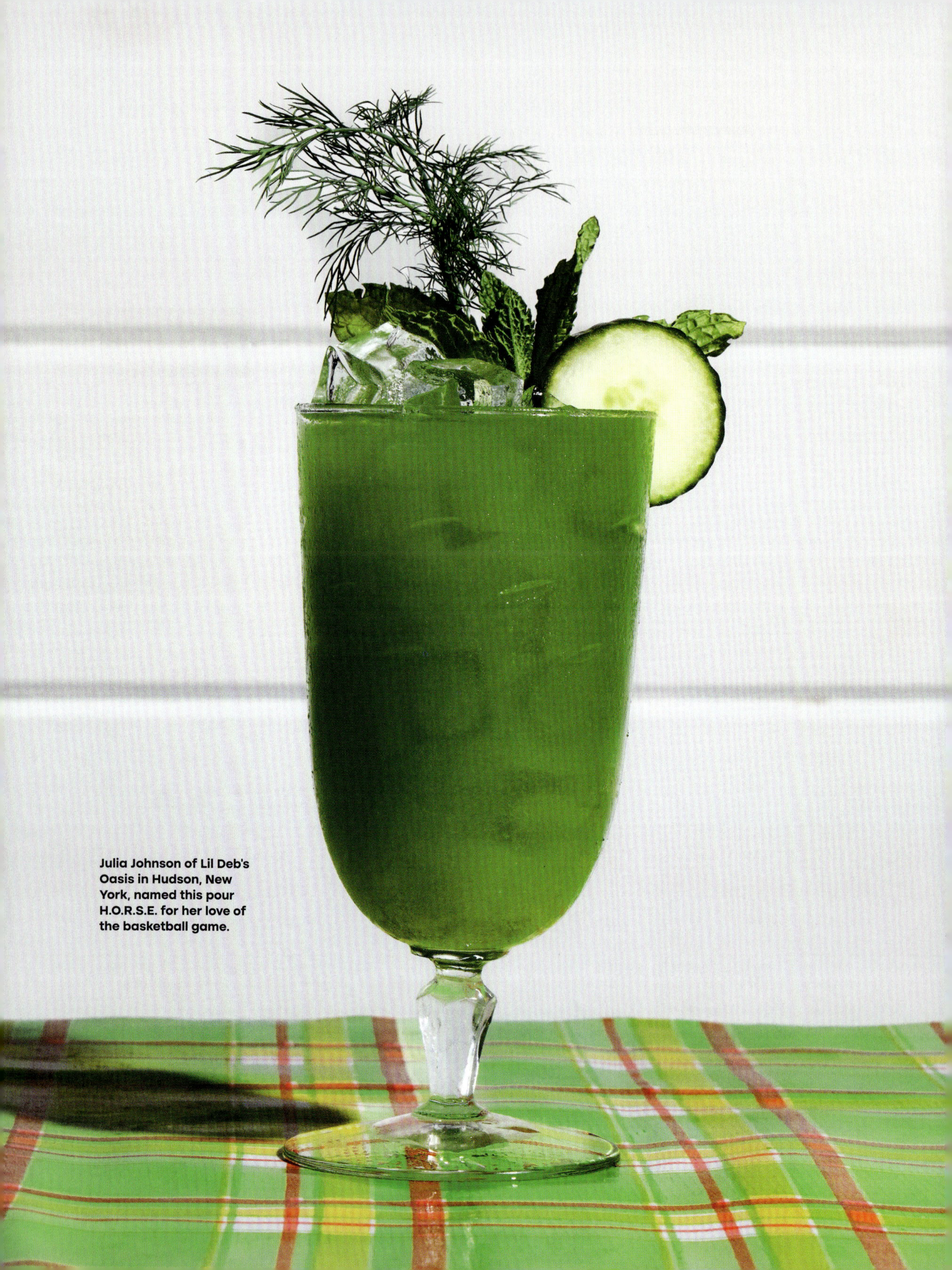
Julia Johnson of Lil Deb's Oasis in Hudson, New York, named this pour H.O.R.S.E. for her love of the basketball game.

 **FLAVOR PROFILE** Think of this spicy sweet pour as a green juice meets a Bloody Mary.

LOW-SUGAR SIPPER!

H.O.R.S.E.

- **2** large cucumbers (about 1½ lbs), peeled and chopped
- **2–3** tsp prepared horseradish, plus more for taste
- **1** cup ice plus more for serving
- **3** Tbsp fresh lime juice, plus more to taste
- **2** Tbsp agave or honey (optional)
- Big pinch of salt, plus more to taste
- Seltzer, chilled, for topping off
- Mint and/or dill for serving, if desired

1 In blender, combine cucumbers, horseradish, 1½ cups cold water, 1 cup ice, lime juice, agave, and salt. Blend until completely smooth.

2 Strain mixture through fine-mesh sieve or cheesecloth into pitcher, pressing the solids to extract all the liquid.

3 Chill mixture about 30 minutes to 1 hour, then taste and adjust salt, lime, or sweetener if needed. Serve over ice in wineglass. Top with seltzer for a spritzy texture. Garnish with cucumber, mint, and/or dill, if desired.

Serves about 6. Per serving: About 34 cal, 0 g fat, (0 g sat fat), 0 mg chol, 65 mg sodium, 7 g carb, 0 g fiber, 6 g sugar, (5 g added sugar), 0.5 g pro

Lip Stain

- **2** beets, roughly chopped
- **1** apple, roughly chopped
- **1** oz Sumac Simple Syrup (recipe below)
- Ice, for shaking and serving
- Sumac Salt (mix 1 Tbsp salt with 1 Tbsp sumac), for rimming
- Sparkling water, chilled, for topping off

1. In blender, add beets, apple, and enough water so blender is three-quarters full. Blend until smooth, then strain through a cheesecloth-lined fine-mesh sieve. (Add more water if needed.)

2. In shaker, add 2 oz of the beet-apple juice and Sumac Simple Syrup and shake without ice 15 to 30 seconds. Add ice and shake again.

3. Rim a Collins glass with Sumac Salt and add ice. Strain mocktail over ice and top with sparkling water.

Serves 1. Per serving: About 83 cal, 0.3 g fat, (0.08 g sat fat), 0 mg chol, 575 mg sodium, 21 g carb, 0.8 g fiber, 19 g sugar, (16.8 g added sugar), 0.4 g pro

Sumac Simple Syrup

HEAT 1 cup water, 1 cup sugar, and 2 Tbsp ground sumac (plus a pinch of salt and 1 strip lemon zest, if desired) in small saucepan over medium heat. **SIMMER**, stirring to dissolve sugar. Once sugar is fully dissolved and mixture is warmed but not boiling, remove from heat. **STEEP** for 15 to 30 minutes, depending on how strong and tangy you desire. **STRAIN** syrup through fine-mesh sieve or cheesecloth into clean jar or bottle. Cool to room temperature before using or storing. **STORE** in the fridge for up to 6 months. This syrup also tastes delicious in lemonade or tea.

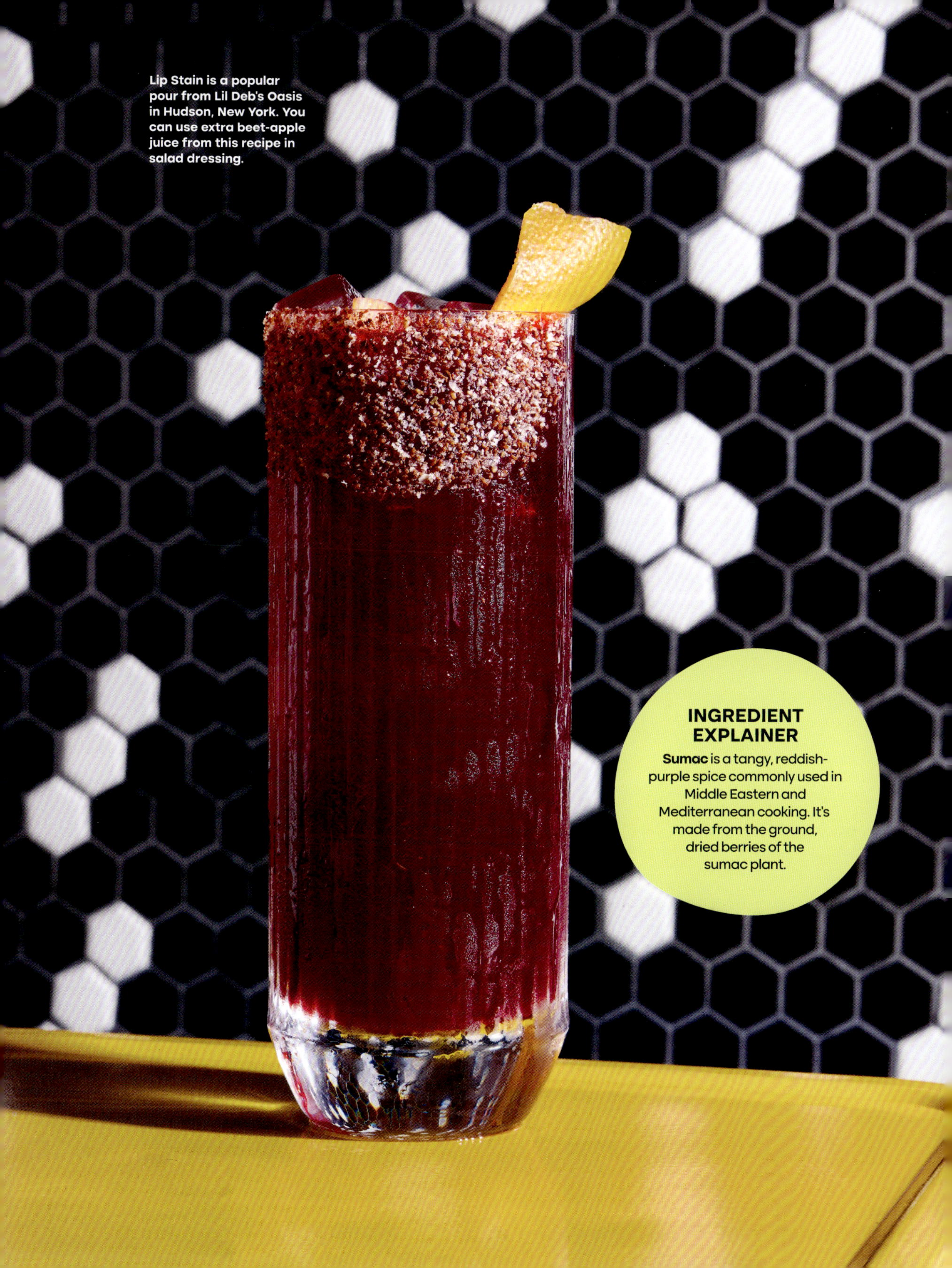

Lip Stain is a popular pour from Lil Deb's Oasis in Hudson, New York. You can use extra beet-apple juice from this recipe in salad dressing.

INGREDIENT EXPLAINER

Sumac is a tangy, reddish-purple spice commonly used in Middle Eastern and Mediterranean cooking. It's made from the ground, dried berries of the sumac plant.

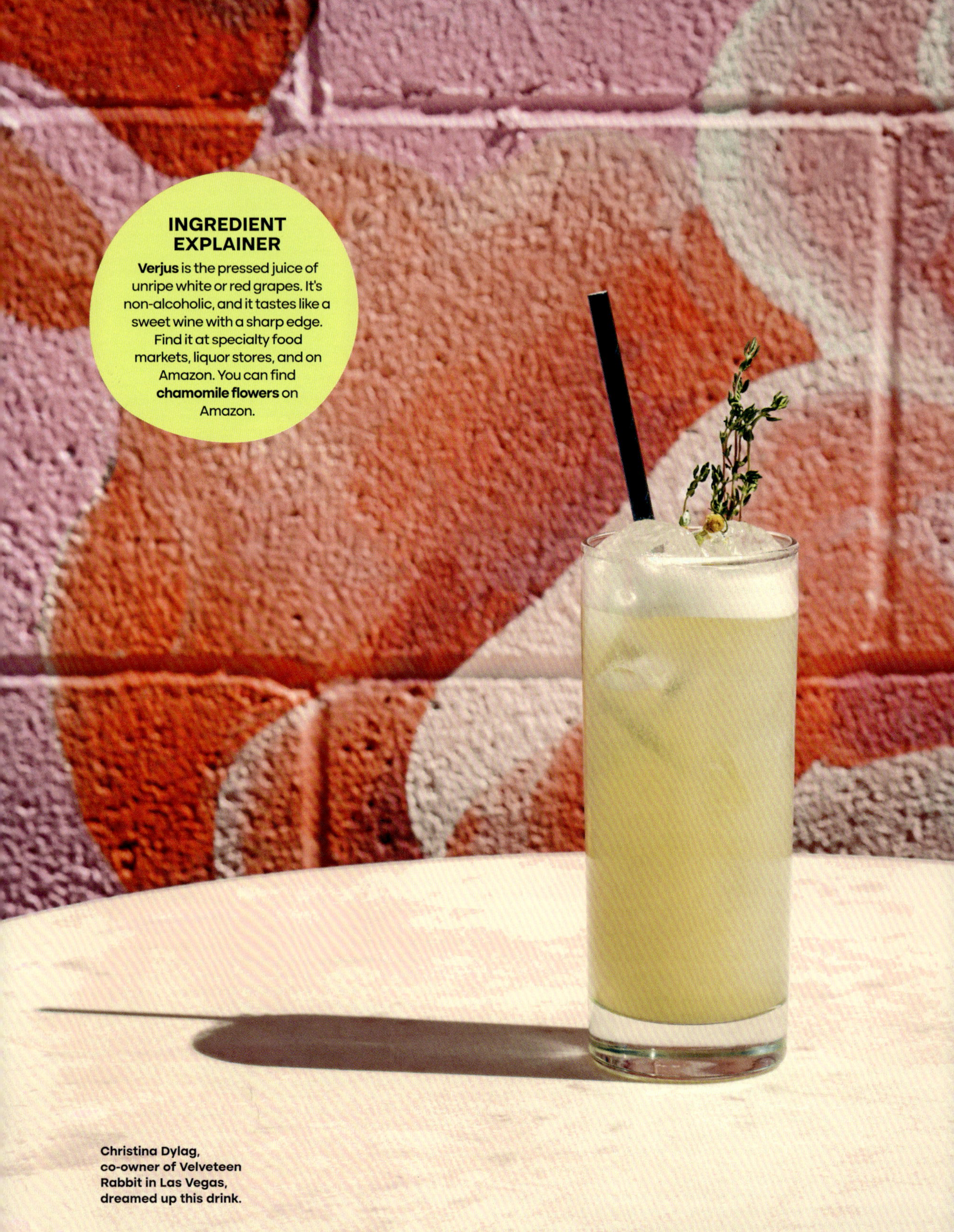

INGREDIENT EXPLAINER

Verjus is the pressed juice of unripe white or red grapes. It's non-alcoholic, and it tastes like a sweet wine with a sharp edge. Find it at specialty food markets, liquor stores, and on Amazon. You can find **chamomile flowers** on Amazon.

Christina Dylag, co-owner of Velveteen Rabbit in Las Vegas, dreamed up this drink.

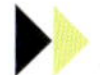

FLAVOR PROFILE This frothy sipper has the creamy tartness of a Ramos gin fizz, the New Orleans cocktail, but with notes of fig and chamomile.

Midnight Idol

- **1** oz white verjus or non-alcoholic white wine
- **1** oz Fig and Chamomile Syrup (recipe below)
- **1** oz coconut milk
- **3/4** oz aquafaba (starchy liquid in a can of chickpeas)
- **1/2** oz lime juice
- Ice, for shaking and serving
- **2** oz tonic water, chilled
- Chamomile flowers and/or thyme sprig, for serving

1. In shaker, add all ingredients (except tonic water and garnishes), and shake 10 to 12 seconds, without ice (known as a dry shake). Add ice and shake for another 10 to 12 seconds (known as a wet shake).
2. Add ice to Collins glass and strain mocktail into glass.
3. Top with tonic water. Garnish with chamomile flowers and thyme sprig.

Serves 1. Per serving: About 181 cal, 6 g fat, (5.3 g sat fat), 0 mg chol, 15.3 mg sodium, 32 g carb, 0.06 g fiber, 29.4 g sugar, (17.4 g added sugar), 1 g pro

Fig and Chamomile Syrup

HEAT 2 cups sugar, 2 cups water, 3 chamomile tea bags, and 1/4 cup fig spread or preserves in medium pot over low/medium for 20 minutes, stirring every few minutes until sugar dissolves. **COOL** and strain through fine-mesh sieve into glass jar. **STORE** in fridge up to a month. For a quick, easy refresher, add a splash to soda water.

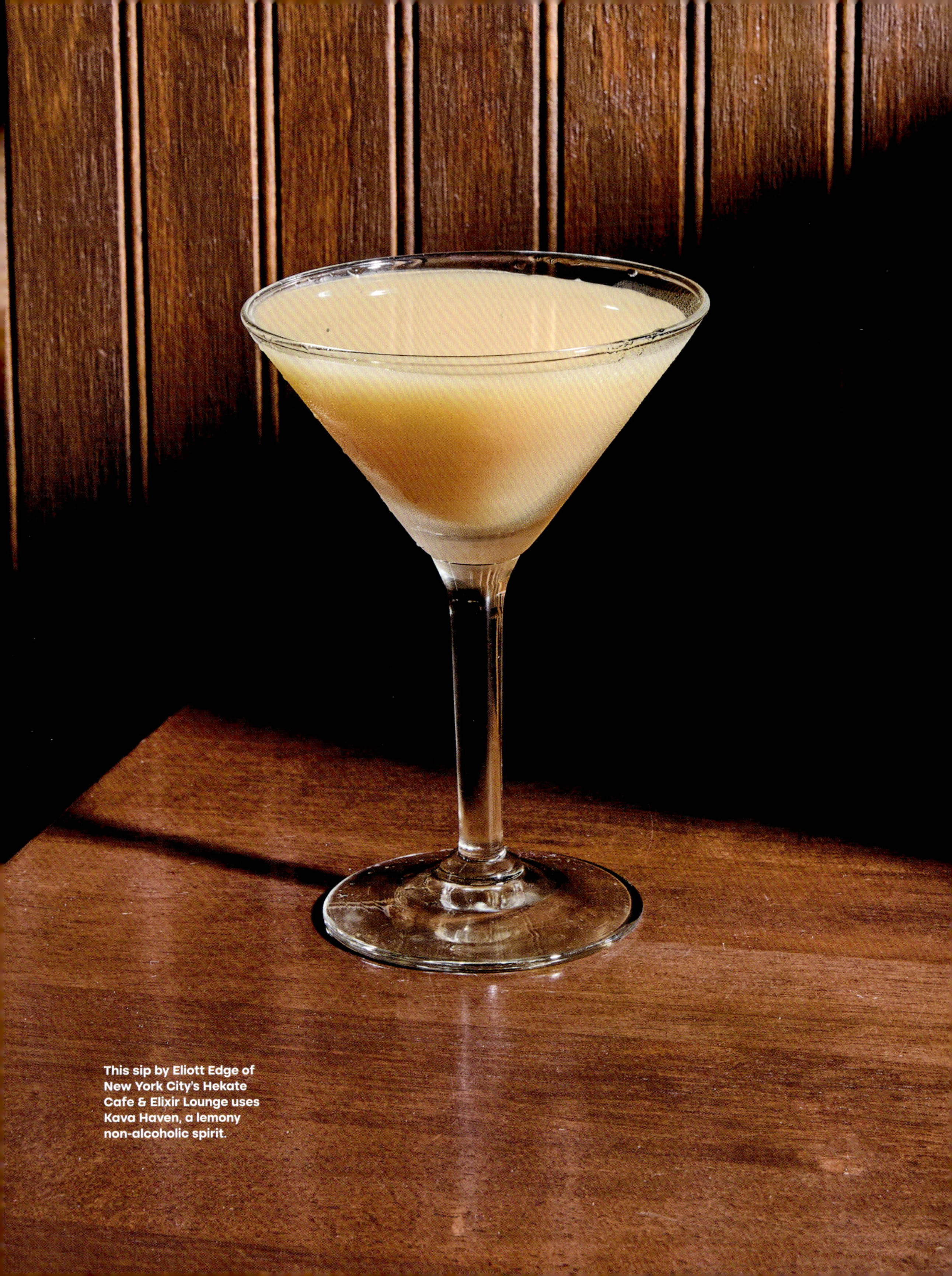

This sip by Eliott Edge of New York City's Hekate Cafe & Elixir Lounge uses Kava Haven, a lemony non-alcoholic spirit.

FLAVOR PROFILE This sipper is like a warm fuzzy blanket, with flavors of ginger, cinnamon, and soothing, spiced molasses.

Kava & Chill

- **2** oz Kava Haven
- **1½** oz Three Spirit Nightcap
- **1** oz Sparkplug Syrup (recipe, p. 110)
- Ice, for shaking

In shaker with ice, shake all ingredients until shaker is frosty. Strain into chilled coupe or martini glass.

Serves 1. Per serving: About 132 cal, 0 g fat, (0 g sat fat), 0 mg chol, 7 mg sodium, 31 g carb, 0 g fiber, 30.5 g sugar, (23 g added sugar), 0 g pro

RAISE THE BAR Kava Haven is a spirit-free blend of ginger and citrus with gentle, mellowing effects. It's also delicious straight. **Three Spirit Nightcap** is a woodsy blend of valerian root, hops, and lemon balm, with notes of maple, vanilla, and spice.

FLAVOR PROFILE Similar to an Aperol spritz, this drink is ripe with red fruit, juicy acidity, a touch of spice, and a bittersweet finish.

Bayberry Spritz

- **1** oz Three Spirit Livener
- **1** oz red verjus (such as Fusion)
- **3/4** oz Giffard Aperitif Bitter
- **1** tsp Simple Syrup With Fresh Bay Leaves (recipe below)
- Ice, for serving
- Fever Tree tonic water, chilled
- **3** bay leaves skewered on toothpick, for serving

1. Add all ingredients (except tonic water and bay leaves) to wineglass filled with ice. Stir.
2. Top with tonic water and garnish with skewered bay leaves.

Serves 1. Per serving: About 133 cal, 0 g fat, (0 g sat fat), 0 mg chol, 10 mg sodium, 33 g carb, 0 g fiber, 30 g sugar, (29.5 g added sugar), 0 g pro

RAISE THE BAR Three Spirit Livener is a spiced elixir with several herbs including ginseng for a natural lift. Its berry flavor and touch of heat add intrigue to this spritz.

Simple Syrup With Fresh Bay Leaves

BRING 2 cups water to boil. **ADD** 2 cups sugar and stir til dissolved. **ADD** About 1 cup fresh bay leaves. **SIMMER** on low heat for 5 to 10 minutes. **STRAIN** through fine-mesh sieve into jar and allow to cool. **STORE** in the refrigerator for about 1 month.

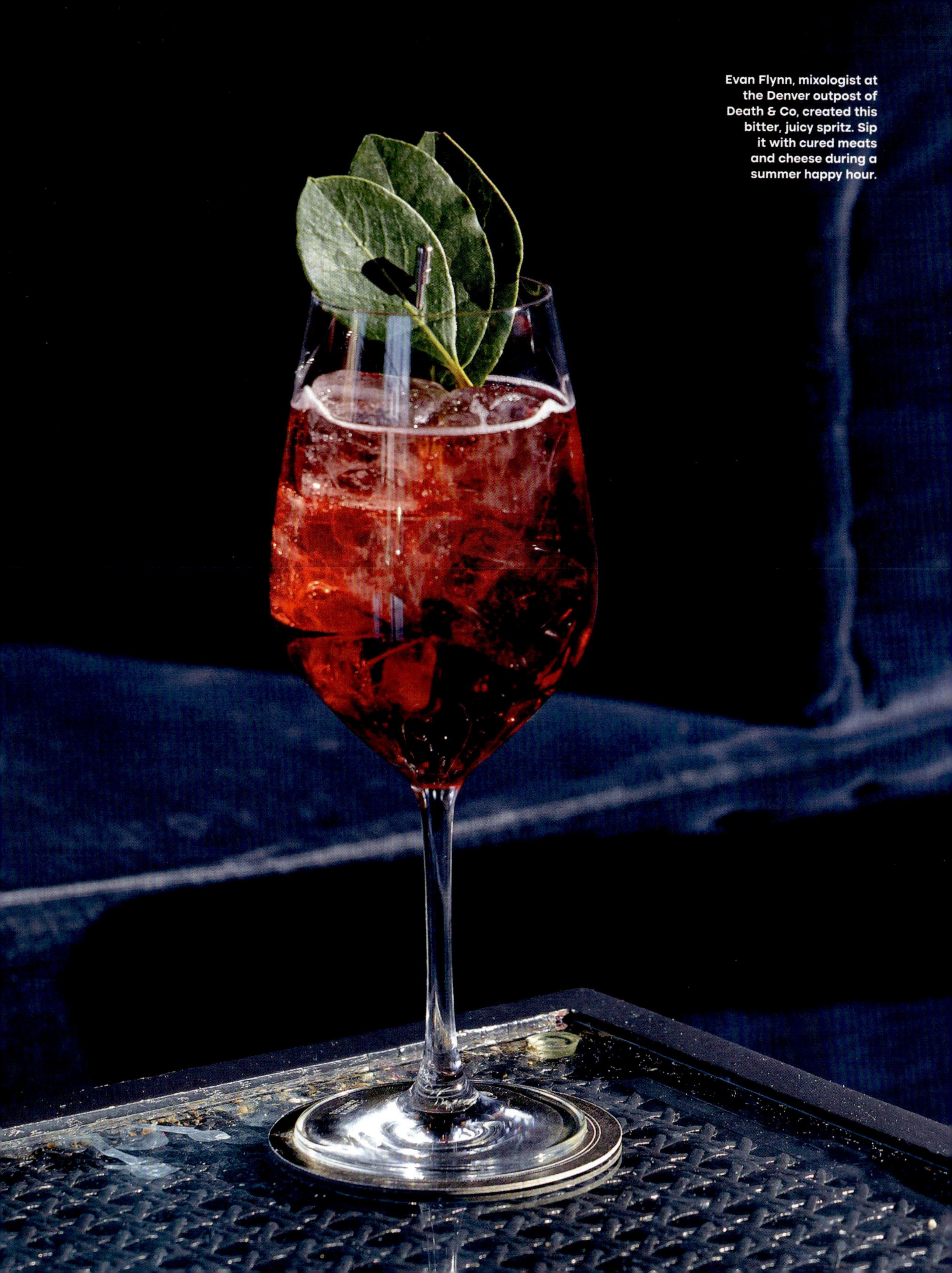

Evan Flynn, mixologist at the Denver outpost of Death & Co, created this bitter, juicy spritz. Sip it with cured meats and cheese during a summer happy hour.

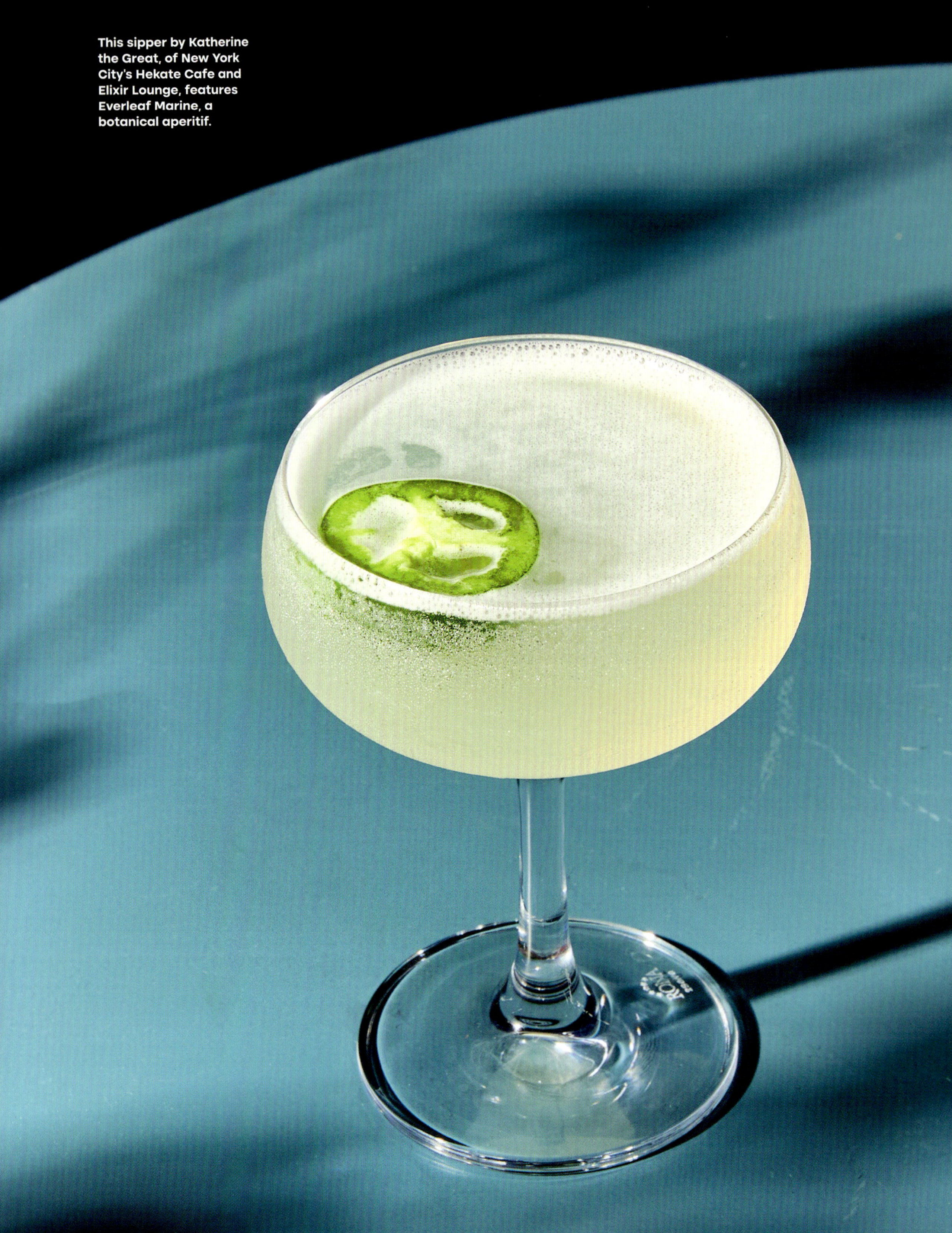

This sipper by Katherine the Great, of New York City's Hekate Cafe and Elixir Lounge, features Everleaf Marine, a botanical aperitif.

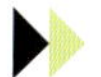

FLAVOR PROFILE Consider this a spicy, crisp, nautical sister to the margarita.

Spicy Seawater

- **2** jalapeño wheels
- **2** oz non-alcoholic tequila (such as Free Spirit)
- **1** oz NA white vermouth (such as Roots Divino Bianco)
- **1** oz Everleaf Marine
- **½** oz Jalapeño Syrup (recipe below)
- **½** oz lime juice
- Ice, for shaking
- Seltzer, chilled, for topping off

1 Muddle 1 jalapeño wheel in shaker. Add all ingredients (except soda water and remaining jalapeño wheel) and ice to shaker. Shake until shaker is frosty.

2 Pour into coupe, top with seltzer, and garnish with remaining jalapeño wheel.

Serves 1. Per serving: About 65 cal, 0 g fat, (0 g sat fat), 0 mg chol, 59 mg sodium, 17 g carb, 0 g fiber, 15.5 g sugar, (15 g added sugar), 0 g pro

RAISE THE BAR White vermouth lifts spritz and aperitif-style cocktails. **Bianco Roots Devino White Vermouth** is herbal and faintly sweet, with notes of rosemary, thyme, and wormwood, the European cousin to sage and tarragon. **Everleaf Marine** is a crisp botanical blend featuring kelp, coastal herbs, and juniper. Enjoy it in a spritz, mojito, marg, or martini, in addition to this recipe.

Jalapeño Syrup

BRING 2 cups water to boil. Add 2 cups sugar and stir until dissolved. Add 2 slices jalapeño. **SIMMER** on low heat for 30 minutes, then let cool. **STRAIN** through fine-mesh sieve into jar.

FLAVOR PROFILE This fusion of faux whiskey and mezcal inspires cozy contemplation.

Hopeless Pyromantic

- **2** oz non-alcoholic whiskey (such as Monday)
- **1** oz The Pathfinder Spirit
- **1** oz NA mezcal or tequila
- **1** oz coconut milk
- **½** oz maple syrup
- **2** dashes Pecan bitters (such as El Guapo Chicory Pecan Bitters)
- Ice, for shaking and serving

In shaker, shake all ingredients and pour into a rocks glass with ice.

Serves 1. Per serving: About 149 cal, 4 g fat, (4 g sat fat), 0 mg chol, 27 mg sodium, 26 g carb, 0 g fiber, 23 g sugar, (22 g added sugar), 0.4 g pro

RAISE THE BAR The Pathfinder Spirit is distilled from hemp and blended with botanicals including wormwood, juniper, saffron, and ginger.

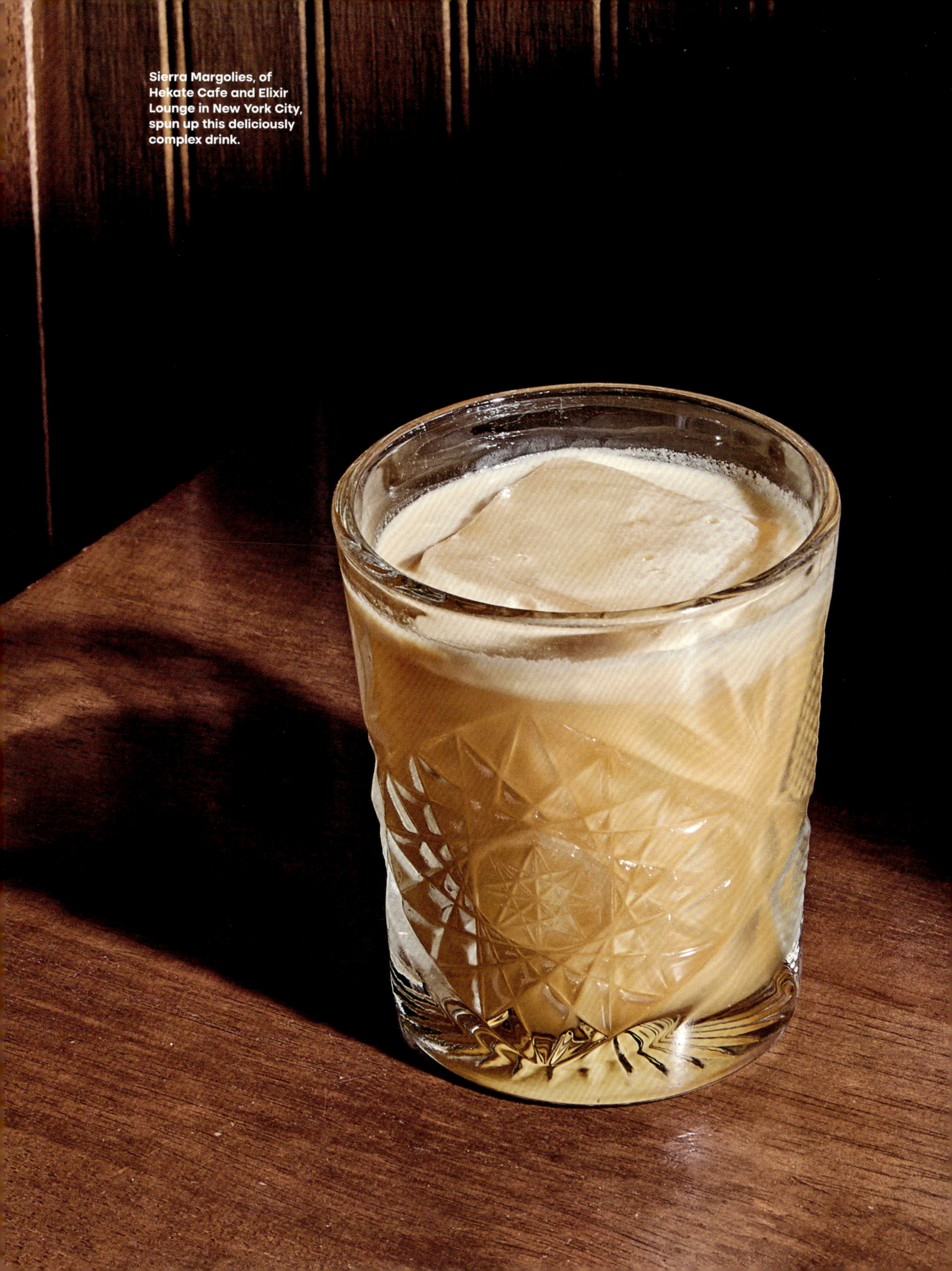

Sierra Margolies, of Hekate Cafe and Elixir Lounge in New York City, spun up this deliciously complex drink.

Celebratory Tipples

Make every holiday a hit.

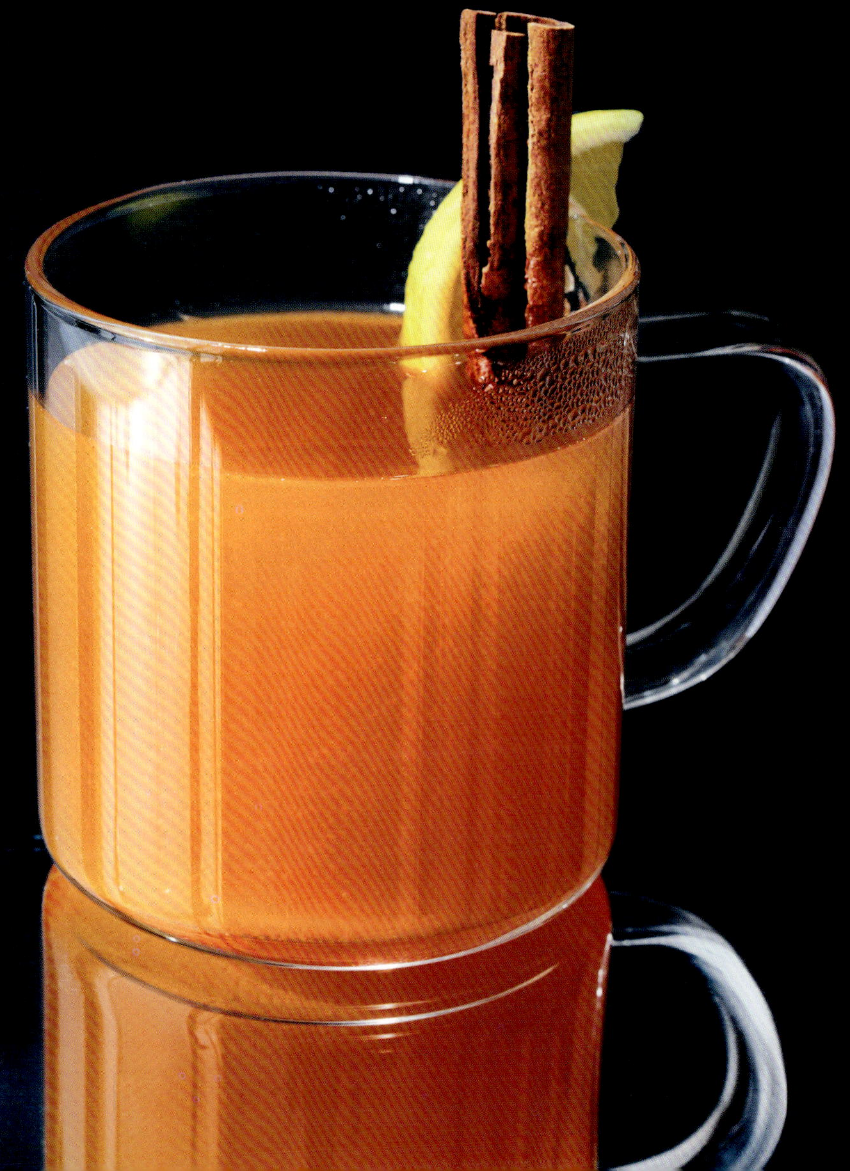

This hot mulled cider warms up any evening between Halloween and New Year's Eve.

Chai Mulled Cider

- **2** cups apple cider
- **2** strips orange zest
- **½** cinnamon stick, plus more for serving, if desired
- **1** tsp black peppercorns
- **4** chai tea bags (such as Twinings)
- Orange or lemon slices, for serving, if desired

1 In small saucepan, combine apple cider, orange zest, cinnamon stick, peppercorns, and ¼ cup water. Bring to a simmer. Remove from heat, add tea bags, and let steep for 5 minutes.

2 Strain cider through fine-mesh sieve into small mugs or teacups. Serve with orange or lemon slices and cinnamon sticks, if desired.

Serves 4. Per serving: About 59 cal, 0 g fat (0 g sat), 0 mg chol, 12 mg sodium, 15 g carb, 0 g fiber, 12 g sugar (0 added sugar), 0 g pro

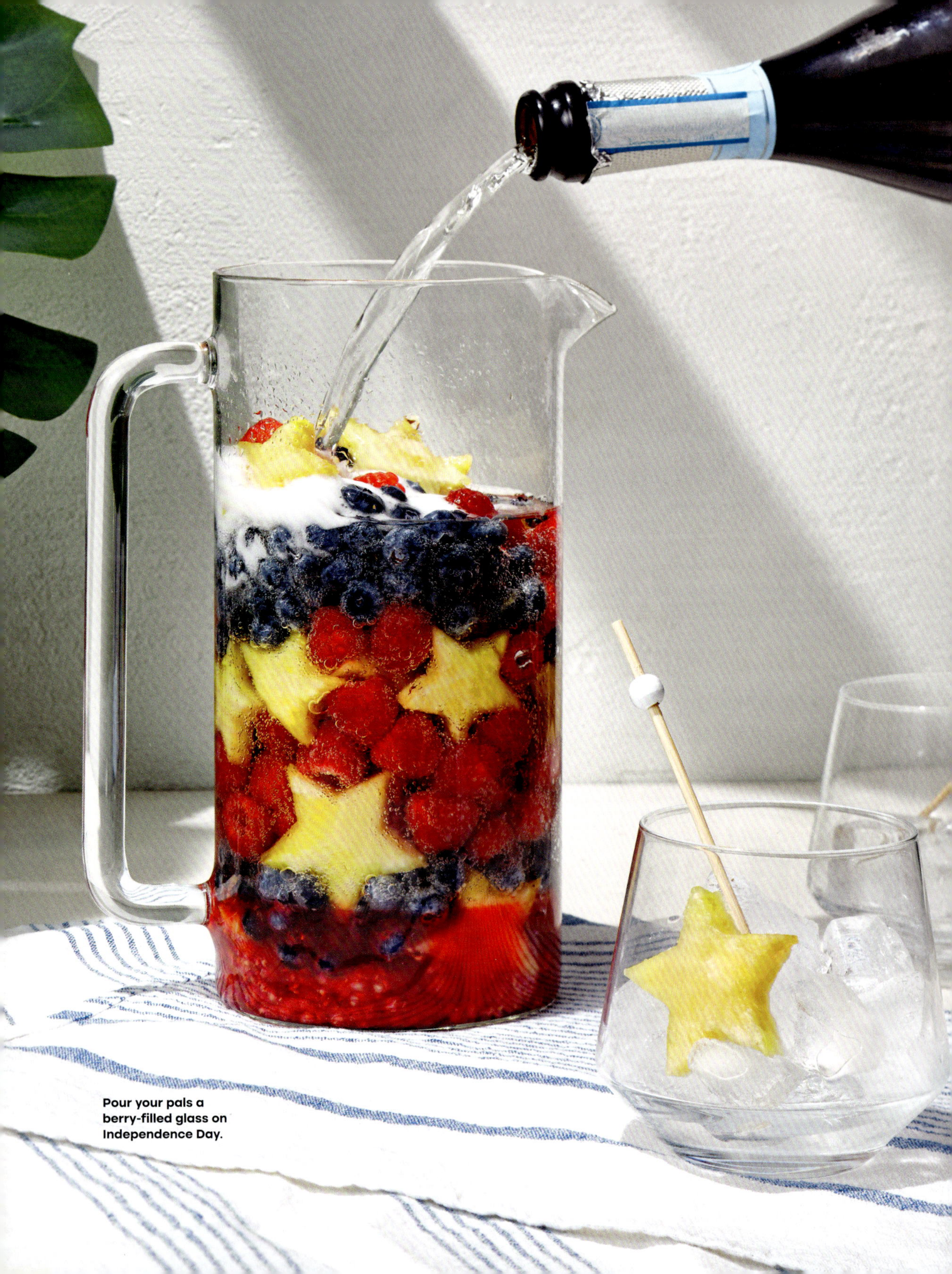

Pour your pals a berry-filled glass on Independence Day.

Star Spangled Spritzer

- **¼** cup sugar
- **2** Tbsp lemon juice
- **4** 6-oz containers raspberries, divided
- **1** pint blueberries
- Pineapple Stars (recipe below)
- **¾** liter sparkling water, chilled
- Ice, for serving

1 In pitcher, muddle sugar, lemon juice, and 1 container raspberries to dissolve sugar.

2 Add blueberries, Pineapple Stars, and remaining raspberries, layering if desired. Add sparkling water. Serve in glasses over ice.

Serves 4 to 6. Per serving: About 143 cal, 1 g fat, (0 g sat fat), 0 mg chol, 34 mg sodium, 36 g carb, 7 g fiber, 26 g sugar, (10 g added sugar), 2 g pro

Pineapple Stars

PEEL pineapple and slice into ¼-inch-thick slices. **USE** small star-shaped cookie cutter to cut out star-shaped pieces. (This works with melons, too!)

Black Charcoal Lemonade

- ¾ cup sugar
- 1 Tbsp activated black charcoal
- 1½ cups fresh lemon juice
- Ice, for serving
- Lemon drops and black candies on toothpick, for serving, if desired

1 In small saucepan, combine sugar and ¾ cup water and bring to a boil. Reduce heat and simmer (do not stir) until sugar dissolves, 3 to 4 minutes. Remove from heat, stir in charcoal, and let cool completely.

2 In large pitcher, combine lemon juice, cooled syrup, and 4 cups water. Serve in ice-filled glasses. Garnish with lemon drops and black candies, if desired.

Serves 6. Per serving: About 111 cal, 0 g fat, (0 g sat fat), 0 mg chol, 5 mg sodium, 29 g carb, 0 g fiber, 27 g sugar, (25 g added sugar), 0 g pro

INGREDIENT EXPLAINER

Activated black charcoal adds drama to drinks. It's made by heating coconut shells, hardwoods, bamboo, or other carbon-rich materials to create a fine powder. It lends an inky hue and a slightly earthy, mineral flavor—perfect for moody sippers like this Halloween-worthy pour. Find food-grade activated black charcoal on Amazon or at Walmart.

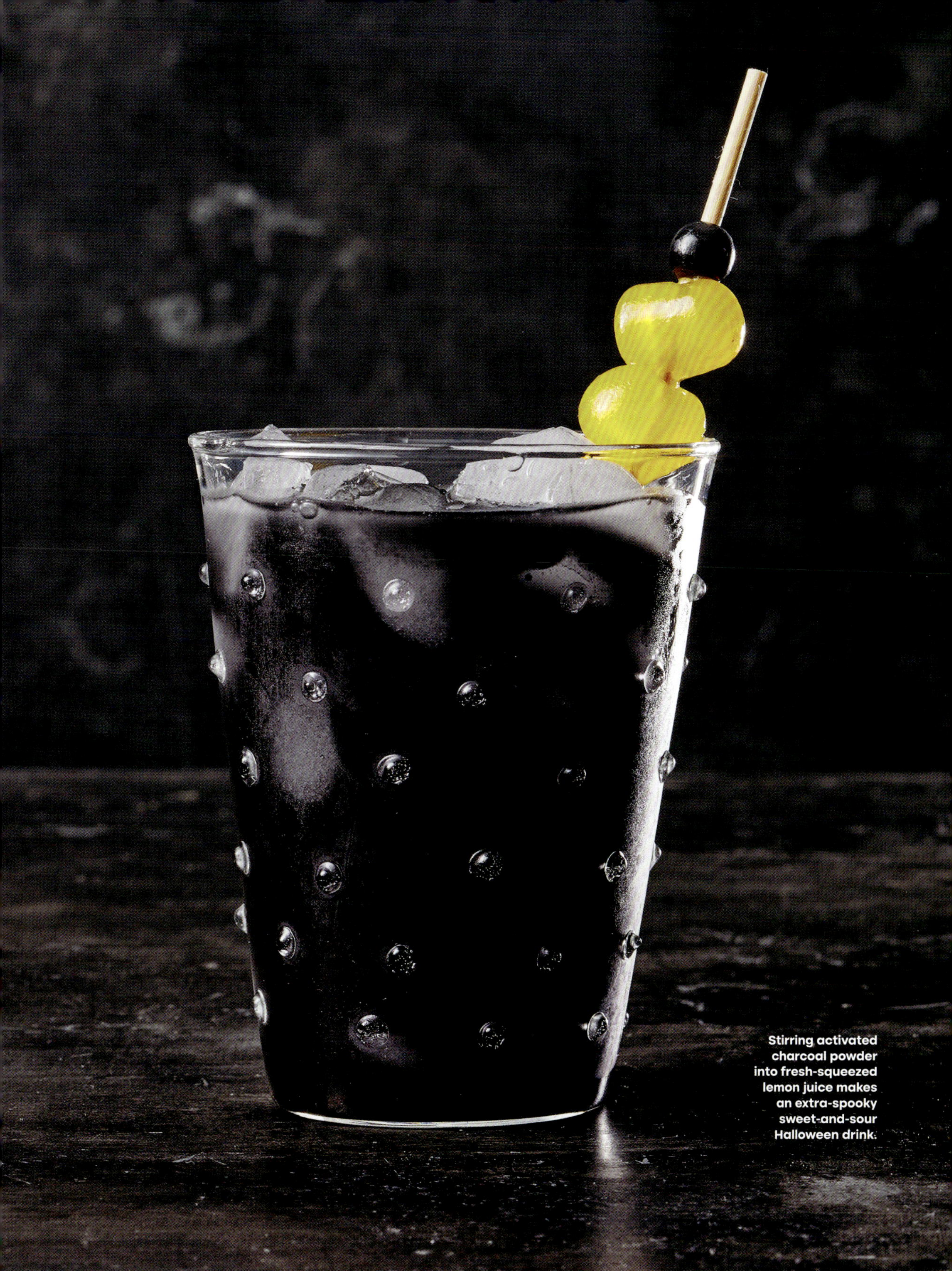

Stirring activated charcoal powder into fresh-squeezed lemon juice makes an extra-spooky sweet-and-sour Halloween drink.

Peach Blossom

- 1⅓ oz peach nectar
- ½ oz non-alcoholic elderflower liqueur (such as Giffard Elderflower)
- ¾ oz citric acid or fresh lemon juice
- Ice, for shaking and serving
- Grapefruit soda, chilled, for serving
- Grapefruit slice and rosemary sprig, for serving

1. In shaker with ice, combine peach nectar, elderflower liqueur, and citric acid. Shake briefly to chill.
2. Strain into ice-filled glass. Top with grapefruit soda.
3. Garnish with a lightly torched grapefruit slice and rosemary sprig.

Serves 1. Per serving: About 106 cal, 0.4 g fat, (0 g sat fat), 0 mg chol, 10.5 mg sodium, 27 g carb, 0 g fiber, 26 g sugar, (12 g added sugar), 0 g pro

INGREDIENT EXPLAINER

Citric acid is the pure, crystalline form of the tangy compound found in citrus fruits. In mocktails, it adds sharp, clean acidity without extra liquid or dilution. It makes flavors pop and mimics the mouthwatering bite of lemon or lime. You can find food-grade citric acid at Walmart or on Amazon.

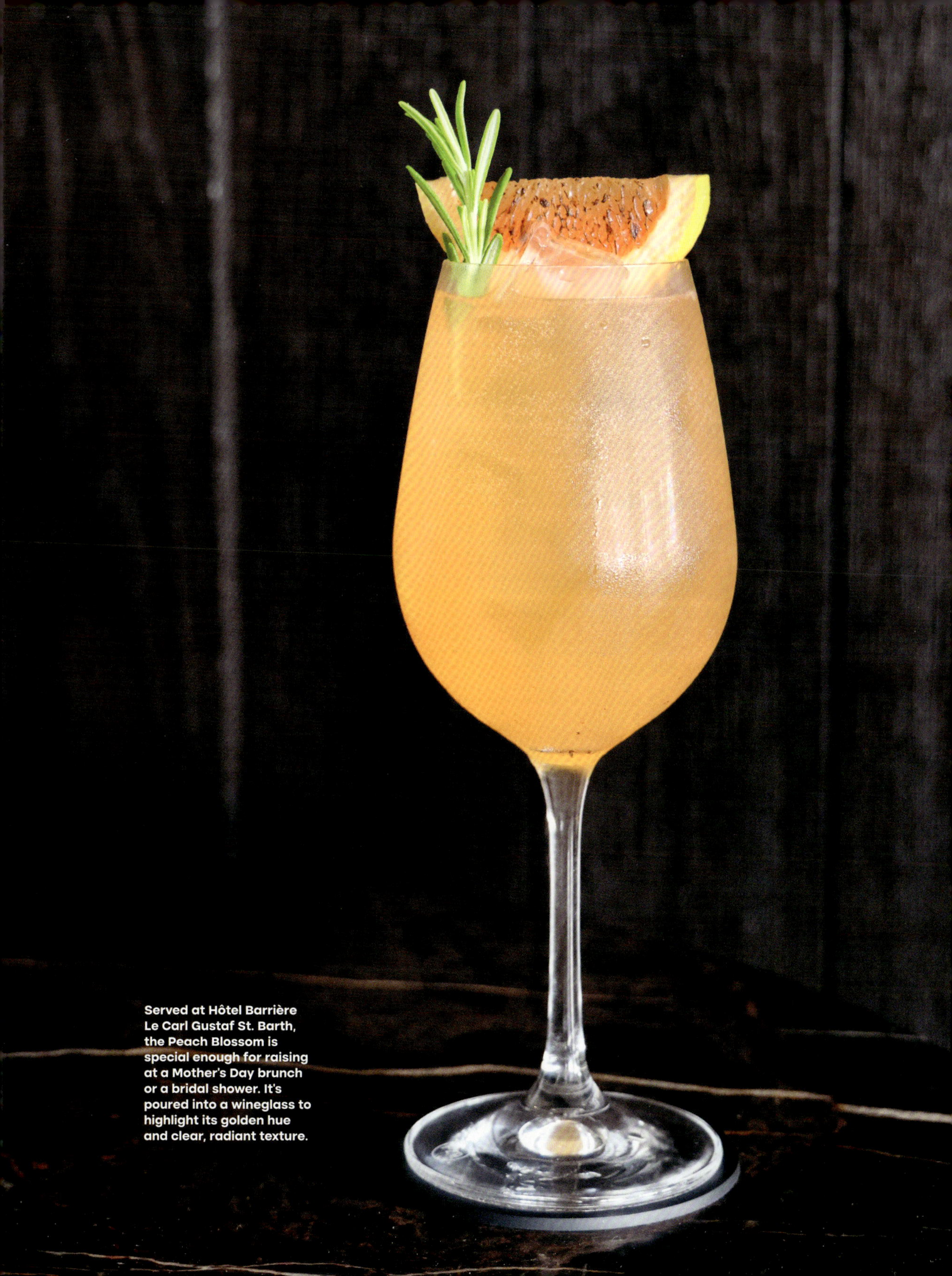

Served at Hôtel Barrière Le Carl Gustaf St. Barth, the Peach Blossom is special enough for raising at a Mother's Day brunch or a bridal shower. It's poured into a wineglass to highlight its golden hue and clear, radiant texture.

Index

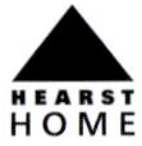

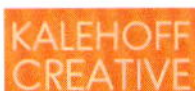

PRODUCED BY KALEHOFF CREATIVE, LLC
Laura Kalehoff Editorial Director
Patrick Crowley Creative Director
Rebecca Kimmons Bell Photo Director
Ray Bass Editor/Researcher
Jo Ann Liguori Copy Editor
Jy Murphy Researcher
Antonina Smith Nutrition Analyst
Jay Krieder Indexer

Library of Congress Cataloging-in-Publication Data
Available on Request
10 9 8 7 6 5 4 3 2 1

Published by Hearst Home, an imprint of
Hearst Books/Hearst Magazine Media, Inc.
300 W 57th Street
New York, NY 10019

For information about custom editions, special sales, premium and corporate purchases: hearst.com/magazines/hearst-books

Printed in China
978-1-958395-70-7

WOMEN'S HEALTH RECIPES + NUTRITION ADVICE
Level up your health with nutrition guides, healthy recipes and so much more. womenshealthmag.com/food

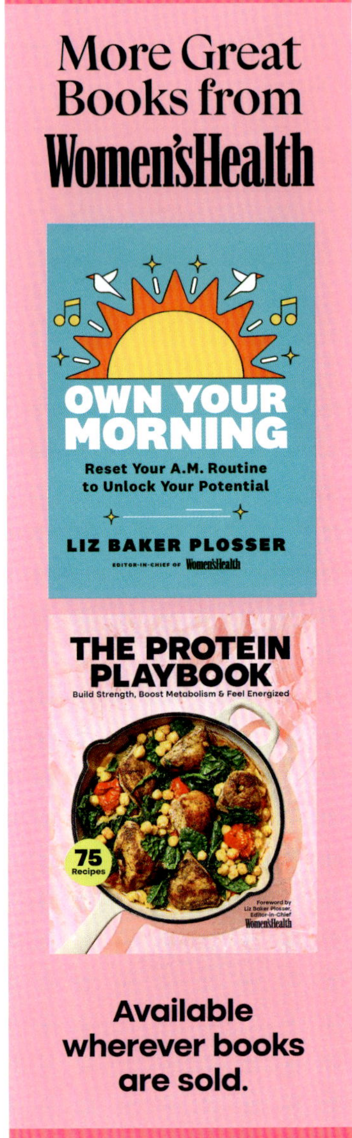

WRITING CREDITS: **SABRINA TALBERT AND ANDI BREITOWICH** (9–11), **EMILY J. SHIFFER** (11), **KATIE BEROHN** (12), **ERIN STROUT** (15–17), **CAITLIN CARLSON** (18), **HALEY WEISS** (21–23), **OLIVIA LUPPINO** (25–27), **TAWNY LARA** (28–31).

PHOTO CREDITS: **CHELSIE CRAIG** (COVER, 44, 46, 67, 69, 70, 96, 101, BACK COVER), **MIRAGEC/GETTY IMAGES** (1) **MAREN CARUSO/GETTY IMAGES** (6), **GETTY IMAGES** (32, 33, 34, 142-143), **ANDREA D'AGOSTO** (2, 4, 42, 57, 64, 74, 117), **ANNA BLAZHUK/GETTY IMAGES** (8, 24), **NIKOLAY POPOV/GETTY IMAGES** (10), **JARREN VINK** (13, 20, 22), **MUTHARDMAN/GETTY IMAGES** (14), **DBENITOSTOCK/GETTY IMAGES** (14), **IRYNA VEKLICH/GETTY IMAGES** (16), **NUGROHO RIDHO/GETTY IMAGES** (19), **TATIANA LAVROVA/GETTY IMAGES** (26), **TIM MORRIS/TRUNK ARCHIVE** (29), **EMILIJA MANEVSKA/GETTY IMAGES** (30), **5PH/GETTY IMAGES** (35), **COURTESY OF BRANDS** (36), **CAGKANSAYIN/GETTY IMAGES** (38), **RAUL RIPNU/500PX/GETTY IMAGES** (40), **JUSTIN STEELE/STUDIO D** (41), **MIKE GARTEN** (48, 51, 53, 54, 73, 102, 136, 139), **TARA DONNE** (58, 119, 120, 123, BACK COVER), **GABY J PHOTOGRAPHY** (60, 81, 124, BACK COVER), **COURTESY OF HÔTEL BARRIÈRE LE CARL GUSTAF ST BARTH** (63, 141), **SAM HANNA** (82), **SHAWN CAMPBELL** (84, 108, 129), **VINCENT BOLOGNINI** (87), **PAH CREATIVE** (91), **LEA GOLIS** (92), **JAMESON KIMBALL AT FAIRMONT BREAKERS LONG BEACH** (95), **JESSE THOMPSON/GETTY IMAGES** (98, BACK COVER), **CHELSEA KYLE/TRUNK ARCHIVE** (105), **JOSH MCDONALD** (106), **JULIA GARTLAND** (76, 88, 111, 114, 126, 130, 133, BACK COVER), **COURTESY OF SUNRIVER RESORT** (112), **DAVID MALOSH** (134).